"Very few contemporary writers in the world of psychotherapy have the foresight to imagine new ways of understanding the human condition, let alone bring these ideas to life in a collection as dynamic and accessible as these. Manu Bazzano is one of these few, and the ideas presented collated by him, and written here by an incredibly interesting selection of writers says a lot about just how important Affect Theory is to understanding our ways of being, and how necessary it is for all of to recognise the subtlety of the Affect which we all engage within, often without knowing it."

Dwight Turner, *activist, writer and public speaker on issues of race, difference and intersectionality in counselling and psychotherapy, UK*

"Within the emergent field created by this book, it is shown how affect in therapy transforms both client and therapist. With clarity and depth, the text illuminates how shared atmospheres, positionality, and embodiment shape the tangible, shifting, and potent exchanges that define a relational therapeutic practice born at the point of contact, extending beyond I–Thou."

Parvy Palmou, *Gestalt therapist, Gender Affirmative Care and Founder of Athenian Gestalt, Greece*

"Richly woven, this is a book to read beyond what is expressed through words. It invites us to follow the signs that point to the felt senses unfolding as we read it, and to recognize the permanent flow/movement of meanings that we experience in everyday life and in therapy."

Salvador Moreno-López, *humanistic-experiential psychotherapist and writer, Mexico*

"*The Primacy of Affect* edited by Manu Bazzano provides its readers with a thorough understanding and insight into the topic. The book introduces a multi-dimensional, new, and complex approach, such that draws from many fields of thought. It also remains attuned to the complex state of affairs of the human sciences discourse."

Noam Israeli, *reader in philosophy and existential therapist, Israel*

The Primacy of Affect

This edited volume features a diverse, eclectic range of voices exploring affect theory in relation to psychotherapy, culture and philosophy.

The 1990s saw the beginning of the affective turn, an important cultural shift which influenced to a considerable degree the arts, politics and culture in general but failed to reach the world of psychotherapy. What would it be like if practices such as psychotherapy took more fully on board the importance of affect? Based on the outcome of a series of seminars led by Manu Bazzano over the course of 2020–2025, this edited volume aims to break new ground by drawing on affect theory, queer and feminist theory, literature and art to outline new ways of practicing psychotherapy and supervision, of doing research and of engaging more creatively and effectively with the political challenges of our time.

The Primacy of Affect: Psychotherapy, Culture, Philosophy will benefit anyone working within or interested in psychotherapy, psychoanalysis, critical theory, contemporary philosophy, politics, the arts and literature.

Manu Bazzano is an author, psychotherapist, Zen teacher and Butoh dancer. He is the founder of *Affect Therapy*. He is a visiting tutor at Cambridge University. His latest book is *Difference and Multiplicity: Adventures in Philosophy and Psychotherapy*.

The Primacy of Affect

Psychotherapy, Culture, Philosophy

Edited by
Manu Bazzano

Routledge
Taylor & Francis Group
LONDON AND NEW YORK

Designed cover image: Getty Images

First published 2027
by Routledge
4 Park Square, Milton Park, Abingdon, Oxon OX14 4RN

and by Routledge
605 Third Avenue, New York, NY 10158

Routledge is an imprint of the Taylor & Francis Group, an informa business

British Library Cataloguing-in-Publication Data
A catalogue record for this book is available from the British Library

ISBN: 978-1-041-13460-2 (hbk)
ISBN: 978-1-041-13459-6 (pbk)
ISBN: 978-1-003-66990-6 (ebk)

DOI: 10.4324/9781003669906

Typeset in Times New Roman
by codeMantra

For Anastasios

Contents

Contributors

Richard Barker is a counsellor and life coach in Port Elizabeth, South Africa.

Manu Bazzano is an author, psychotherapist, Zen teacher and Butoh dancer. He is the founder of *Affect Therapy*. He is a visiting tutor at Cambridge University. His latest book is *Difference and Multiplicity: Adventures in Philosophy and Psychotherapy.*

Emily Corrie is a psychotherapist in private practice trained in the existential school but has found her home outside. She runs an organic farm in France where she spends a lot of her time weeding onions.

Dr. Anastasios Gaitanidis is a relational psychoanalyst in private practice. In addition to his clinical work as a psychoanalyst, he has held appointments as a senior lecturer and Director of Studies and provided clinical and research supervision to psychotherapists and counselling psychologists at Regents, University of Roehampton and Metanoia. He currently holds the position of Visiting Professor for the DPsych in Counselling Psychology at Regent's University London. He is the theory editor of the *European Journal of Psychotherapy and Counselling* and an author who has published a substantial body of academic work, including journal articles and edited books over the years, with a recent book publication entitled *The Sublime in Everyday Life*.

Seb Heid works as a person-centred therapist in London. He came into counselling after previous lives, first in academia (PhD in Phonetics) and then in industry (software engineer). Driven by a lifelong passion for philosophy, he is specifically interested in the phenomenology of power, theory of affect, the understanding of understanding and the intersections of all of these themes in the task of making sense of our postmodern existence, philosophically and as a practitioner relating to the struggles of his clients. Born and educated in Germany, he has lived in the United Kingdom for more than 25 years now.

Margarita Karkagianni was born in Athens. She has studied Political Sciences (1994, Panteion University, BA) and Social and Political Thought (1996, University of Warwick, MA). She completed her PhD in Philosophy at the Centre for Modern European Philosophy at the University of Kingston. Her PhD thesis title is "Nuance and tension: A study of Bergson's idea of intensity." In 2022, she completed her postdoctoral research in the Department of Political Science and Public Administration at the National and Kapodistrian University of Athens. Her postdoctoral research concerned the problem of time in Nietzsche, Bergson and Benjamin. She is currently completing a monograph on the problem of time and the critique of modernity in Nietzsche, Bergson and Benjamin. Her main publications concern the philosophy of time, memory and experience in Bergson, Benjamin and Baudelaire, Deleuze's theory of temporality, the problem of time and the concept of genealogy in Nietzsche and Bergson, the concept of politics and the "political" in Deleuze and Nietzsche.

Zoë Krupka is a writer, academic, psychotherapist and supervisor working in Melbourne, Australia. She currently lectures and supervises research in the Master of Counselling and Psychotherapy and Psychology programmes at The Cairnmillar Institute. Her current research interests include anti-oppressive supervision practice and critical conceptual interrogations of burnout and trauma. You can find a full collection of media publications at www.zoekrupka.com, academic publications on ResearchGate and Zoe in the kitchen at parties.

Nikolaos Kypriotakis has studied Physics (where he reads Physics as a kind of philosophy) and has been trained in person-centred and focusing-oriented psychotherapy, in person-centred supervision and in children focusing. Currently, he works as a focusing trainer in the Hellenic Focusing Center (HFC). He is a coordinator for The International Focusing Institute (TIFI), New York. He co-edited in English (together with Judy Moore) the two-volume publication *Senses of Focusing* (Athens, 2021; https://sensesoffocusing.weebly.com). He has also translated Gendlin's seminal text, *Focusing*, into Greek (published 2023), and he is currently writing, in Greek, a comprehensive book on Focusing (theory and applications) that will be published in 2025–26. He was the editor-in-chief of the magazine *Εποχή-Epoché* (*Phenomenological Psychotherapies*), for the issues n.1 to n.16 (former subtitle: *Psychotherapy, Phenomenology, Hermeneutics*). For two years, he was the General Secretary of the Hellenic Association for the Person-Centered and Experiential Approach (HAPCEA).

Glenn Nicholls is a psychotherapist, supervisor, trainer, executive coach and organizational development consultant. He has a private practice in Cambridge and London and currently leads an integrative supervision training in Central London. Nietzsche has had a profound influence on his personal development as a psychotherapist.

Agniya Pasechnik-Lyle is a humanistic psychologist and certified hypnotherapist with an MSc in Psychology and a PhD candidate at HSE University. Her doctoral research examines *Encounter in Everyday Life*, focusing on how encounters can be utilized as tools for self-help, emotional balance and personal transformation. As a research fellow at the Laboratory of Creativity, she co-developed the educational programme *PICK* (Plurilingual Intercultural Creative Key), which promotes creativity and emotional maturity through an interdisciplinary framework. With significant experience working with artists and other creative professionals, she brings a nuanced understanding of how affective and symbolic processes facilitate personal growth. Her work on *Encounter* highlights its accessibility and potential to foster meaning, joy and self-awareness in everyday life.

Yannis Rigas is practising person-centred and focusing-oriented psychotherapy. As an independent researcher, he is interested in process-philosophy, drawing on thinkers such as Deleuze, Guattari, Braidotti, Whitehead, Massumi and Gendlin, and this interest extends into published essays and public seminars on critical posthumanism, media studies, architecture, queer theory and practice, and critical psychoanalysis. Yannis is also translating works by Deleuze, Guattari and related theorists into Greek. The whole of this attempt is to help rendering this theory practical and accessible, grounding it in everyday ethical practices that promote existential and collective joyful symbiosis, preserving the life's complexity by avoiding any reduction to dogmas or market-driven products.

Michalis Tegos is a postdoctoral researcher in the Department of Philosophy at the University of Ioannina, Greece.

Konstantinos Tzikas is a psychotherapist, translator and author based in Athens, Greece. Trained in person-centred and focusing-oriented psychotherapy, he also serves as an assistant facilitator of an LGBTQI+ existential therapy group. His previous studies include English Literature (BA and MA, National and Kapodistrian University of Athens), Media Studies (BA, Panteion University of Social and Political Sciences) and Gender Studies (MA, Panteion). He formerly worked as a journalist for various publications and has contributed articles and book reviews. He is the author of one collection of short stories and has translated two books into English.

Dániel Ványi is an independent researcher and a psychological counsellor from Budapest, Hungary. He has an MA degree in Social Psychology, and he is a certified person-centred counsellor. He has published academic articles in the fields of critical social psychology and psychotherapy in Hungarian and English. He has practised and studied meditation for more than 15 years with various teachers and Buddhism-inspired meditation groups. He is interested in the interconnections between philosophy, politics, therapeutic practice and meditation.

Introduction

Manu Bazzano

Partly reflecting the conversations that took place during a series of seminars I have given on the topic between 2020 and 2025, this book tackles Affect and its implications/applications in the fields of psychotherapy, culture, and philosophy.

Affect is the term that contemporary philosophy, inspired by Spinoza, gave to the intensity of life itself, *before* it collides with the prism of subjectivity and becomes translated into individual emotions, feelings, and thoughts. Deleuze, Massumi, and other thinkers discussed in these pages helped restore affect from its reduction to subjective emotion. Affect followed a similar trajectory to the one travelled over centuries by the Greek term *ψῦχή* (psyche): from Heraclitus' expansive notion in fragment 35, where it is depicted as limitless and way beyond the human domain, to an atomized entity wedged within the individual psychic apparatus and even brain – often a disembodied brain.

Each in its own way, the following contributions attempt to problematize and redescribe affect, partly by restoring its forgotten, expansive nature. Whether discussing dreamwork, supervision, or therapy, whether tracing the presence of affect in key counter-traditional philosophical texts or searching for therapeutic responses outside the sleepy, acquiescent practices of the mainstream, the collective endeavour on display in the pages that follow gazes towards a new horizon. It aspires to an expansive view that may help enliven therapy, culture, and the practice of philosophy.

*

What would it mean to pay closer attention to affect as a pre-personal phenomenon, *before* its reduction to subjective feelings, thoughts, and emotions? What would it mean to include within the exploration of the latter (mainstream psychotherapy's main preoccupation) a more comprehensive investigation of how individual feelings, thoughts, and responses come about?

The 1990s saw the beginning of the affective turn, an important cultural shift that influenced to a considerable degree the arts, politics, and culture in general but failed to reach the world of psychotherapy. The affective turn was important, and its effects are still felt today. It signalled the end of the 'language turn'. What would it be like if practices such as psychotherapy take more fully on board the

DOI: 10.4324/9781003669906-1

importance of affect? And what are the implications of bringing this perspective to the examination of culture in general?

Drawing on affect theory, queer and feminist theory, literature, and art, this book breaks new ground by outlining new ways of practising psychotherapy and supervision, of doing research and of engaging more creatively and effectively with the political challenges of our time.

What would it mean to take a fresh look at some key cultural and psychological notions such as relatedness, research, dreams, sexuality, gender, identity, and politics? The common theme emerging from the chapters in this book is a nudge towards a decentring of the self – not by evading the self and its ever-present claims but by embedding it in a wider field. This wider field *includes* the relational domain, the in-between but crucially goes beyond it – not necessarily towards spiritual transcendence (one of the ways in which the widening of the field of attention and research may happen) but within a field of *immanence*, entirely within this impermanent world of phenomena we inhabit.

I hope readers will be affected by this book; that they will in turn find ways to activate the particular inspiration or provocation they may have found in these pages, and that they will be motivated to experiment further and create new horizons in their life and work.

Manu Bazzano, London, 18 January 2026

Chapter 1

What is Affect Therapy?

Manu Bazzano

Affect therapy

Affect Therapy is a new approach to therapy that I began to assemble in 2020 via regular online and hybrid seminars, as well as through ongoing research and study. It is still a work in progress. This chapter reflects the development so far. As a result of the lively conversations with participants to the seminars (many of them keen like myself to find a way out of a tired and mechanical way of practising therapy even before the advent of AI), a clear set of theoretical directions and connections has emerged. The question often being asked is: how do you apply these exciting ideas in practice? In the past, I have been prone to countering this sort of question with a facetious remark, labelling it as a sign of philistine pragmatism. I would invite the interlocutor to hold the ideas lightly in their mind, to absorb them and let them percolate until they may begin to alter the way one relates to a patient/client, and more generally perceive and understand what is actually happening in the therapy room. I later began to wonder if that is enough and gradually became more alert to the need for examples and descriptions that may help get a sense of how affect therapy may look in practice. However, it is important to remember that far from claiming ultimate truths on any matter, theory is at heart an attempt to redescribe the world, create new concepts, and alter the map of the field of experience. In that sense, I remain a phenomenologist, and more accurately a post-phenomenologist, in the sense that I refuse to be held captive to phenomenology's persistent entanglement with primitive subjectivism and that I remain doubtful of the scholastic phenomenology routinely taught in psychotherapy trainings.

Bringing affect theory into therapy decentres subjectivity – not merely because it helps us see through the conceited avatars of neoliberal brands such as Positive Psychology or the fatuous miracle cures peddled by self-styled trauma experts dominating the psych world in our time. Applying affect theory to therapy also interrogates and problematizes softer and genuinely progressive incarnations of subjectivism (be they relational, intersubjective, eco-based, spiritually-infused, or politically astute). As an "approach to culture, history, and politics that focuses on the role of prelinguistic or nonlinguistic forces, or affects", affect theory invites us to look at what shapes us, recognizing that we are not Cartesian subjects nor solid

DOI: 10.4324/9781003669906-2

entities but a *coalition of affects* – and that these are "neither under our 'conscious' control nor even necessarily within the register of our awareness—and they can only sometimes be captured in language" (Schaefer, 2016).

Bearing that in mind, I will briefly outline below the salient points that make Affect Therapy. I will start with some theoretical orientation and will then illustrate the way I have used some of its methodologies so far. A more detailed, in-depth descriptions will be found in *The Affect Therapy Manifesto* (Bazzano, forthcoming).

A counter-traditional lineage

Affect Therapy's philosophical framework goes way back: to 500 BC, its starting point being the fragments of the enigmatic philosopher/poet Heraclitus. Not many people may have heard of him, but quite a few will recognize fragment B12: *you can't step in the same river twice.* With his appreciation of becoming, of life-death as process and flux, Heraclitus represents the beginning of the Western counter-tradition (Bazzano & Webb, 2016). Simply put, this is a mode of thought whose manifestations have so far included humanism, scepticism, fideism, as well as the opening of philosophy and psychology to poetry and the arts. Despite the supremacy of the *tradition* (initiated by Platonism) within philosophy, the humanities, and mainstream culture through the centuries, the counter-tradition continues to afford inspiration and visionary insights through its errant lineage. It has resisted the hyper-rationalization and institutionalization of culture typical of the tradition, offering the semblance of a home for heretics of all sorts.

The twice-heretic 17th-century philosopher Spinoza is a case in point. His astonishing, still controversial phrase *Deus sive Natura* – God or Nature – continues to affirm materialism *and* spirituality, something nearly incomprehensible to the tradition in whose binary modes of thinking we are mostly entangled. Spinoza's view of nature is the very foundation of Affect Therapy. Nature is for him "a life no longer lived on the basis of need, in terms of means and ends, but according to a production, a *productivity*, a potency, in terms of causes and effects" (Deleuze, 1988, p.3, emphasis added). Productivity here means turning passive forces into active ones. It means activating power within oneself – power no longer understood in the delusional and reactive sense of domination over a fellow human being – *potestas* –but as active creation – *potentia.*

It implies a movement from *being affected* to *affecting* – a movement of active *creation*, be it aesthetic in the Foucauldian sense of care of self, or existential in the Sartrean sense of self-creation. It may also be understood in terms of what Nietzsche calls, in the preface to the second edition of his *Gay Science*, great health, an active transformation of illness:

> Only great pain, that long, slow pain that takes its time and in which we are burned, as it were, over green wood, forces us philosophers to descend into our

> ultimate depths and put aside all trust, everything good-natured, veiling, mild, average - things in which formerly we may have found our humanity.
>
> (Nietzsche, 2001, p.6)

What is counter-traditional in Spinoza's and Nietzsche's perspectives is their affirmation of life. Spinoza's *sad passions* – sadness, hatred, contempt, desolation, spite, guilt, and so on – are lenses through which our perception of life becomes distorted and as a result we tend to denigrate life itself. Anticipating Nietzsche, Spinoza stresses that the aim of the philosopher is to become free and to be able to affirm life. One way to do this is by transforming the sad passions into active, affirming forces. As with Nietzsche's texts, Spinoza's words are affecting, instilling in the reader a determination (what he calls *conatus*, a will to live and thrive) to *act* and take further what has affected us rather than remaining passive recipients of a set of ideas or circumstances. This is how their respective philosophy becomes alive and fulfils its power as potential. Rather than signposts of a mummified canon, these pointers are provocations to act, to become more of what one is and can be, remembering that in order to do that, we mustn't have the faintest notion of who we are.

Affect theory, as I understand it (for it is a multifaceted phenomenon with different interpretations), capitalized on the counter-tradition and, in particular, those expressions that followed in the wake of Spinoza, Nietzsche, and others – that flowering of thought, particularly in France during the 1970s, that came to be arbitrarily labelled poststructuralism.

Deleuze, in particular, has performed the remarkable task of rewriting Spinoza's work (as well as Leibniz, Nietzsche, and Bergson) making it pliable to a necessary project of emancipatory ethics that pivots around notions of power, useful as a way to introduce an examination of Affect Therapy's methodologies.

Power as creative *potentia* is a positive force when we allow it to do its thing. When we do not, it becomes *potestas*, the need to dominate others in order to cover up our own sense of inferiority. Blatant manifestations of potestas are on display on the world stage as we speak – reactionary and fascistic politics based on fear of otherness paired with asinine attitudes to life, love, and work. Potestas is driven by malice, Deleuze teaches us; it wants to prevent someone from doing what they can do, to express their *potentia*. Power is in itself not bad; it often becomes twisted and malicious when we don't exercise it creatively and choose instead to act as tin-pot dictators whether in our home or in the seats of power. Having potestas does not bring real joy. Real joy comes from the exertion of potentia – to allow our creative powers their full range (Deleuze, 1988). This is not an easy task; it involves, Nietzsche would say, a certain degree of struggle so as to gain mastery – not over others, but over the means needed for our particular expression in the world – words for the writer, colour for the painter, the body itself for the dancer, hands for the healer, wisdom, and compassion for the teacher. This mastery is what brings real joy.

Affect Therapy in practice

The aim of Affect Therapy is joy. Holding lightly some of the ideas outlined above, let us now have a closer look at aspects of affect therapy in practice.

Working with the enigmatic message

A banal yet still popular idea holds that when learning within a psychoanalytic/psychodynamic frame, we focus on the patient/client's childhood, whereas if training within humanistic/existential modalities, we concentrate on the here and now. The first mode is an invitation for the archaeologists among us to dig in the hope of finding the alleged original cause of the person's current predicament. The second mode asks us to be present in the new-age abstract platitude of the here and now. Affect Therapy does not bypass the past. How can we? How can the past (or the future) be erased from the present? The past is right here.

Why would anyone wish to bypass the useful insights inherited from psychoanalysis and naively maintain that what you see is what you get? More to the point, Affect Therapy does not discard the unconscious – it redescribes it. It does not accept canonical interpretations – be they within the object relations model, trauma-informed therapy, or attachment theory. Redescribing the unconscious implies questioning how it has been commonly understood, including (a) something that needs to be sanitized and/or made conscious; (b) a foundational ground of being; and (c) a set of signifiers that can be decoded within a language structure.

Redescribing the unconscious means placing it somewhere else entirely: Laplanche (1998) placed it inside the *enigmatic message* unwittingly implanted by parents or primary caregivers in the infant (Bazzano, 2023a). Neither the parent nor the infant is consciously aware of this transmission, but it is nevertheless felt by the infant. As with all adults, parents are not themselves conscious of the mysterious life they carry within them – a life that the infant dimly perceives via the parent's bodily presence. Yet the unconscious kernel of what the parent exudes via their embodied sexuality, their dreamworld, their unspecified aspirations, and so on, deeply influences the child. While remaining largely indecipherable, the enigmatic message we carry within us from infancy can be indirectly, tentatively felt. The enigmatic message *is* the unconscious – the alien within us, the entity whose bulk, breadth, and flush give depth and meaning to our existence, provided we can *activate* it, by turning its passively felt manifestation within us into the general purpose of our life. This is when the enigmatic message we inherited turns into our own cultural message to the world.

In therapy, this scenario constitutes the backdrop, the therapist's invisible compass that may guide her through the labyrinth of the patient's psyche. On some occasions, the backdrop comes to the fore. The client may be speaking of their felt experience of their mother or father. The therapist may then ask: "What was the general feel of your parents' presence as you were growing up? And if you were to condense it into a message, a phrase, a statement, what would that be? How is it felt at this moment?" These questions are approximations, mere jottings of my own experiments when responding to clients whose exploration spontaneously veers towards their experience of their parents' impact on them.

Whether the enigmatic message is perceived as positive or negative, nurturing or neglectful, encouraging or disheartening, and supportive or abusive, what matters is being able to activate it in some way, so as to allow the person to experience more fully their power (*potentia*). As with affect itself, the enigmatic message remains indecipherable; it is not made conscious, as the positivist dictates of our age has it, but is activated, and by activating it, we begin to trace our own path. We don't have to know before we act, nor accept facticity either as fate or attempt to evade it through fantasy. Instead, we can *invent* our response to the given, Sartre might say. This could be described within an ontology of actuality. For affect therapy, the task is to turn a passive affect into an active one. The enigmatic message remains unknown, yet activating its tangible effect initiates a process of transformation. Any therapeutic work that shuns this crucial movement is bound to remain incomplete.

Zen

Enigma is also a key word in Zen, particularly within those aspects of the tradition where the influence of Ch'an – the indigenous form of Chinese Buddhism infused with Taoism – is particularly felt.

Offshoots of contemplative practices have in recent years been incorporated into the world of therapy – noticeably mindfulness and transpersonal psychology. I have written on both mindfulness (e.g., Bazzano, 2013, 2014, 2016a, 2019b) and transpersonal psychology (e.g., Bazzano, 2016b, 2017). Here, I will focus on three aspects of the one contemplative tradition that is wholly in accord with Affect Therapy: *Zen.*

(a) The first aspect deals directly with affect. Zen is firmly rooted in the practice of silent meditation (*zazen*) honed and refined through several social cultural, mythological, and spiritual hues and contexts – from India to China to Vietnam, Korea, and in the 12th century to Japan, where it became known as Zen and was subsequently transmitted to the Western Hemisphere. As Zen practitioners, we wear these layers on our skin. When participating in a *sesshin* (a traditional retreat), I wear closest to my body a Japanese *jubon* (lightweight kimono); the middle layer is a Chinese *koromo*, and the outer layer is the Indian *kesa*, a rectangular, patched vestment draped over the shoulder. A piece of clothing is not just a piece of clothing. We may see it as inanimate, but nothing is inanimate. If we can afford to be affected, a piece of clothing can break our heart open as we wear it. Traditionally, the kesa, the outer garment (as its lay version, a patched bib-like garment worn on one's neck), is made of layers of discarded cloth that may at times carry a particular meaning. My dharma brother Jeremy Ryōkan Woodcock had sewn in his kesa a shred cut from the shirt of a dear friend who had passed away. "Tradition" takes on a wholly different meaning from what we normally mean by it: no longer obeisance to a mummified canon but a current of affect that runs through many generations.

By the simple act of taking the posture of zazen, we enter a live stream that has been running for centuries and continues to flow into the future as we breathe. To practise Zen is to lay our bodymind open to being affected beyond our comprehension. It is to invite the long dead, the living, and those waiting to be born to the austere banquet of our silent contemplation. It is to lay ourselves open to the 10,000 things, to all phenomena of this ephemeral and mysterious world, each of them with something to teach us if we are open to listen.

(b) The second aspect has to do with what Dōgen, the 13th-century Japanese monk, writer, and founder of the Sōtō school of Zen, memorably calls *imperceptible mutual aid*. The emphasis in Dōgen shifts away from awareness and the self's conscious striving, focusing instead on what is "unknowable to human consciousness" (Waddell & Abe, 2002, p.12n). When practising together with genuine intent, we support one another in ways that are often subtle, invisible, and beyond our conscious perception. After the initial conscious resolve to sit in zazen, practice unfolds by itself when we are able to step aside and refrain from ascribing a goal dictated by the ego-self's projects.

In the words of Waddell and Abe (2002, p.13n):

> Samadhi [meditative absorption] is not dead stillness without perception or consciousness; the mind (perception and consciousness) of the zazen practicer and its environment (the sphere of the mind) arise and subside but do so within the realm of the jijuyū samadhi, in which the practicer is one with all things, so this does not result in any disturbance.

It may sound paradoxical to ears trained in the philosophical Western tradition: the natural emergence of wisdom (*prajna*) in meditation practice does not belong to the domain of human agency. This and other aspects of dharma teachings sound paradoxical because we normally choose to focus on consciousness and conscious effort. On these matters, our era is the era of the hypertrophy of consciousness – witness the focus on conscious effort in most mindfulness approaches to therapy, or the virtual disappearance of the unconscious in contemporary psychotherapy's discourse, including psychodynamic therapy.

(c) The third aspect has to do with the notion, prevalent in Ch'an Buddhism, of the *Dark-Enigma*. According to the 9th-century Ch'an master Qingyuan Weixin, there are three stages in the understanding of the dharma: in the first stage, we see mountains as mountains and rivers as rivers; in the second, mountains are no longer mountains and rivers are no longer rivers; in the third stage, we see mountains as mountains and rivers as rivers (Weixin, 1990). The second stage is essential. I wouldn't want to pass judgement on other spiritual traditions, systems of thought, and even psychotherapy orientations, but it might not be entirely wrong to say that foundational concepts within most of them are confirmed and fortified at every stage of learning. The Zen tradition is unusual in encouraging doubt, perplexity, and disorientation as fundamental to the training. This is even more striking in

Ch'an: "Once we are oriented – David Hinton writes – the next step is disorientation", and this, he goes on to say, is "the Ch'an wrecking-crew most fundamental methodology: the dismantling of our conceptual orientation" (2020, p.90).

The dismantling of concepts, kissing goodbye to metaphysics, and other marvellous constructions is essential to glimpsing our original nature, often described as Buddha-nature, Buddha-mind, prajna-wisdom. Trying to name the unnameable, Lao-Tzu named it dark-enigma. Lin-Chi (Rinzai) spoke of the "dark enigma of all Buddhas" and referred to the Dharma as "dark enigma in quiet mystery" (Hinton, 2020, p.93). Dark-enigma – and dark-enigma learning – effortlessly harmonizes with the notion of affect as described so far. It denotes a vital move to a prelinguistic domain where the division between consciousness and empirical reality becomes blurred. As with affect, dark-enigma cannot be represented explicitly but only hinted at. It can only be recognized through direct experience even though it is possible to hint at the core of this experience – as countless Zen haikus and sayings from the old masters have done. Ultimately, the experience of dark-enigma – as with the experience of turning the sad affects into affirmation – points to freedom. In the words of the Ch'an master Kuo Hsiang: "No-mind inhabits the mystery of things… There, you can know dark-enigmas extent. There, your movements range free" (Hinton, 2020, p.93).

Daimonology

Despite its superficial championing of difference and plurality, contemporary culture and psychology rest on the belief in a self-existing entity called "the individual". But there can be no real championing of difference without an understanding of the inherently composite nature of the self. There can be no real appreciation of difference in others without an appreciation of our own originary multiplicity. Arguably, this goes against the very foundations of psychology, an endeavour whose entire *raison d'être* rests on the shaky construct of a human indivisible (*in-dividual*) core, a notion that conventional psychotherapy has eagerly embraced.

We are not individuals but dividuals; not a solid, self-existing entity but a coalition of affects. In antiquity, this was reflected in the main polytheistic religions, some of which survive to this day. But a belief in many gods does not automatically extend to the plurality of the psyche. The contemporary view of human psychology remains decisively monotheistic. It has failed to take on board the insights from quantum theory, believing instead in "soul atomism" (Nietzsche, 1978, p.25). The self (what some would call "soul") is an irreducible multiplicity. Its seeming solidity is not attributable to a pre-existing, unchangeable core but to a particular affective tendency that has taken over at a given time in our life, choosing and structuring various micro-dispositions. Nietzsche is very specific about this. He identifies these various affective tendencies as "drives (*Triebe*), desires (*Begierding*), instincts (*Instinkte*), powers (*Mächte*), forces (*Kräfte*), impulses (*Reize*), passions (*Leidenschaften*), feelings (*Gefühlen*) … and pathos (*Pathos*)" (Bazzano, 2019a, p.65). None of these is primal. Nietzsche takes his cue from the 18th-century polymath Boscovich (2015), who spoke of force points – dynamic, differentiate centres within a force field – as an alternative to the alleged unity of the atom.

Psychotherapy did take notice of the multiplicity of the psyche but strived in various ways to marshal their autonomy within an integrated whole. Drawing selectively on Nietzsche, Jung wrote of *personification*, the tendency of psychic contents to take on a distinct personality – only to summarily reduce them to archetypal matrices. Melanie Klein's remarkable discovery of partial objects was similarly reined in to serve the agenda of the primal family sphere thus losing the partial object's fluidity, autonomy, and resistance to being integrated. Humanistic psychology spoke of configurations of self – aspects of the psyche reductively seen as peripheral offshoots of a core entity, the self, forgetting that the self is also one of these configurations. Inspired by William James, the founder of psychosynthesis Roberto Assagioli suggested the notion of sub-personalities, a key feature of his approach albeit understood as useful yet inchoate facets of the psyche in need of a synthesis.

The list could go on. The common trend at work, despite the theoretical differences, is to integrate, rein in, synthesize, and ultimately repress the inherently autonomous nature of the affects. Nietzsche's perspective remains vital in affect therapy. It respects the autonomy of affects; it accepts the risk that comes with a continuous creative struggle between various drives, instincts, desires, and so on without capitulating to the notion of an atomistic self at the centre of it all.

My Zen teacher at the time, Genpo Roshi, developed Big Mind, a method that capitalized on a technique called voice dialogue, in turn inspired by Jung's personification. I started to use it in my work 23 years ago as I had found it to be an expedient way to give permission whether working with a person or a group to allow their different "voices" – be they anger, desire, sadness, joy, grief, etc. – to speak freely with as little mediation and/or censorship as possible. However, I soon realized there was a twofold agenda in the Big Mind model. Not only did the voices need to be integrated, as the familiar trope in all conventional psychology demands. They also had to be reined it by so-called transpersonal voices such as wisdom, compassion, and big mind. At that point, I moved away from the Big Mind template and started working from a different conjecture. I redescribed "voices" in the Socratic language of the *daimonic*, with one crucial difference: no longer a solitary daimon as in Socrates (a deadly, demanding voice, in my view, who would rather see Socrates sentenced to death than continuing to live) but a host of *daimons* in the plural – unintegrated, complex, and generative, expanding the range of experience through a decentring of the self. I renamed this way of working with affects *daimonology* as a mode that goes counter both integration and organicism. Organicism often features in political and philosophical writings bent on devising a dialectical resolution to the inorganic or non-integrated self, a move made popular by Gramsci's notion of the organic intellectual and against which the philologist and Marxist thinker Sebastiano Timpanaro posited an "interdisciplinary 'extravagance', permitting of self-internal warring factions with no need for dialectical resolution" (Geue, 2025, p.86).

In opposing both integration and organicism, Affect Therapy invites us to an unfettered exploration of affects – of their autonomy and generative powers.

Butoh

Part 3 of Spinoza's *Ethics* discusses the affects. Proposition 2 (1996, p.71) states: "no one has yet determined what the body can do", an affirmation that opened up, mostly as a result of Deleuze's interpretation (1988), a new field of exploration, at variance with the stilted view of the mind ruling over the body. It also engendered a rewriting of the body as a field of potential, affected by other bodies, humans and non-humans (and, I would add, living or dead, animate or inanimate), highlighting at the same time the fluidity of human nature.

This fluid, open-ended perspective on the body was later taken up in a wholly different context by Artaud with his notion of the body without organs, a topic discussed in more detail elsewhere (Bazzano, 2023b), an innovative way to rethink the body outside the confines of metaphysics, medicine, and language. The term was coined by Artaud in his never-to-be aired 1947 radio play *To have done with the judgement of God* (Artaud, 1947), one that deeply influenced one of the founders of butoh, Hijikata. The last passage of this short play reads:

> Man is sick because he is badly constructed. We must make up our minds to strip him bare in order to scrape off that animalcule that itches him mortally, god, and with god his organs. For you can tie me up if you wish, but there is nothing more useless than an organ. When you will have made him a body without organs, then you will have delivered him from all his automatic reactions and restored him to his true freedom. Then you will teach him again to dance wrong-side out as in the frenzy of dance halls and this wrong side out will be his real place.
> (Artaud, 1947)

Of all the movement practices I dabbled with over the years, *butoh* is the one that touched me the most, the one I studied consistently, and the one that deals with the questions posed by Spinoza and Artaud. What's more, it is the closest to Affect Therapy. Butoh is much more than a movement practice. *Ankoku butoh* is also avant-garde theatre, a spiritual practice close to animism, as well as first and foremost a form of *dance*, described by one of his founders, Tatsumi Hijikata, as "gestures buried in the darkness" (Mikami, 2016, p.17).

I first came across butoh in the late 1990s when I attended some workshops with butoh performer and teacher Marie-Gabrielle Rotie, and on one occasion I had the good fortune to participate in a workshop with the great Japanese dancer and choreographer Ko Murobushi. After a long gap and the occasional workshop with other teachers (Horacio Ganem in Berlin and Yumino Seki in the United Kingdom),

I resumed the study and practice of butoh in earnest in 2018 with Rotie. From the following year, I also started putting on a series of solo performances. This came as a surprise to me, and it had to do with two distinct experiences during two separate butoh workshop. The first one was in late October 2020. My friend and colleague Richard Pearce was on my mind throughout that weekend. I had spoken to him during my lunch break and learned that he was in palliative care. It was Halloween, and I walked up and down a muddy path under the constant drizzle as I spoke to him. During our conversation, the sun came out briefly. He told me he had been sent home from the hospital and of his desire, in the time he has left, to bring his work to some sort of completion.

Back to the workshop, the teacher said: "'Listen up. Here's our next exercise'. We're struggling to come back to life. We are dead or getting close to being dead. It's irreversible. But damn it, we want to live, no matter what".

With inexorable winter choking our dreams, we can't help dreaming of spring. We're dying to live, wrenching our frame from the dark earth, struggling to articulate our thirst like a bulb springing up against wind and rain, battered by the same foul weather as Macbeth and on the very same island. Where will I get my strength from? But it must be done. Lying on the cold hard floor, I struggle to get up, honoured and burdened by Richard's request to take up his work. I'm rising from the dead. Or, caught in between life and death, I dig my fingernails into the grimy soil and look up and up at the murky air. Afterwards, Marie-Gabrielle has kind words for all. It's on me, for some reason, that she rests her gaze for a while and says: "everyone did well; but your desperation was real". I am taken aback, I weep quietly, invisibly. And I know it's because of Richard, this savage yearning to rise from the chthonic soil to complete the work and in the process making the existential therapy Richard loved a little less daft, a little less bland, a little less majoritarian – a little less fixated on goals, measurements, and outcomes. I smile at Marie-Gabrielle in gratitude and say nothing. But now I'm laughing at myself. I'm no butoh expert. I haven't a clue. The soft earth will claim me too at some further point. As it claimed Richard, interrupting our conversations, leaving our work incomplete, sending forth shivers of doubt, ripples of agonizing speech and an awful silence. How can I speak from this hollow space? At the same time, do I have a choice? Richard's reply would be a resonant yes. To choose, to act. To choose (Sartrean) freedom, courage, and emancipation was, as I understand it, central to his own personal and political ethos. How can I say it? From words and sounds we emerge, from the dark earth, mother of ghosts and ghouls, we rise from the swarming soil, from the wet muddy chaosmos up and up through mist and rain and it will be dawn again, and spring. Again. *Cool it with a baboon's blood/Then the charm is firm and good.*

*

The second experience occurred during an exercise known in butoh as ash walk (*hokotai*), an experiment in fragility and disappearance, of being moved rather than moving. On this particular occasion, a variation was introduced: instead of walking forward, we were asked to walk backward. As I gazed in front of me, I pictured the past as I was irredeemably moving away from it. It could not be amended; there was nothing I could do but gaze at it while an unmovable force kept pushing me backward. Then, as I continued the slow movement backwards, I remembered: in Paul Klee's painting *Angelus Novus*, Walter Benjamin saw the angel of history, wanting to redeem the past while being swept backwards by a forceful wind that traps his wings, a wind whose name is progress. As I continued to move, tears filled my eyes. I recognized my personal history of pain – heartbreak, grief, and loss blending with the larger agony of history itself – the nightmare of wars, injustices, and genocides.

Butoh has become integral to my Affect Therapy workshops and Zen retreats. The backward ash walk in particular continues to have a strong impact on participants and constitutes a source of inspiration to them. I find butoh beneficial in other ways, including the expression through movement of affects in my daimonology work.

The dream rhizome and affect-based supervision and research

Affect therapy is evolving as we speak. At present, there are three more aspects to the work: the dream rhizome, affect-based supervision, and affect-based research. All of these are discussed in three separate chapters in the present book.

The dream rhizome builds on Gordon Lawrence's social dreaming matrix and is grounded on the notion of the dream as affect in visual attire. I have found affect-based supervision, particularly group supervision, to be a stimulating experiment in redirecting the focus of the inquiry to the wider field surrounding the client and their content, thus escaping the crude subjectivism that is the main feature of conventional therapy.

As for affect-based research, it makes the most of post-qualitative research, away from the limitations of quantitative research and the sentimental platitudes of qualitative research.

As with the other experiments discussed in this chapter, these last three forms of inquiry point towards a new horizon of possibilities for working within the domains of psyche, experience, and thought.

References

Artaud, A. (1947) *To have done with the Judgment of God* https://www.surrealism-plays.com/Artaud.html retrieved 06 Dec 2025.

Bazzano, M. (2013) 'In Praise of Stress Induction: Mindfulness Revisited', *European Journal of Psychotherapy and Counselling*, Vol. 15, pp. 174–185, https://doi.org/10.1080/13642537.2013.793474.

Bazzano, M. (Ed) (2014) *After Mindfulness: New Perspectives on Psychology and Meditation*. London: Palgrave McMillan.

Bazzano, M. & Webb, J. (2016) *Therapy and the Counter-tradition: The Edge of Philosophy*. Abingdon, OX: Routledge.

Bazzano, M. (2016a) 'The Fourth Treasure: Psychotherapy's Contribution to the Dharma', in R. Purser, D. Forbes, & A. Burke (eds) *Handbook of Mindfulness: Culture, Context and Social Engagement*. New York: Springer, pp. 293–304.

Bazzano, M. (2016b) 'House of Cards: On Ken Wilber's Neo-Traditionalism', *Self & Society,* Vol. 44, No. 2, pp. 145–156, https://doi.org/10.1080/03060497.2016.1147666.
Bazzano, M. (2017) 'Why Zen is not Transpersonal', in M. Bazzano (ed) *Zen and Therapy: Heretical Perspectives*. Abingdon, OX: Routledge, 80–94.
Bazzano, M. (2019a) *Nietzsche and Psychotherapy.* Abingdon, OX: Routledge.
Bazzano, M. (2019b) 'Meditation and the Post-Secular Condition', *Psychotherapy and Politics International*, Vol. 17, No. 2. https://onlinelibrary.wiley.com/doi/abs/10.1002/ppi.1490.
Bazzano, M. (2023a) 'Where It Was, the Other Shall Be', in M. Bazzano (ed) *Subversion and Desire: Pathways to Transindividuation.* Abingdon, OX: Routledge, pp. 39–58.
Bazzano, M. (2023b) 'What Is the Body?', in M. Bazzano (ed) *Subversion and Desire: Pathways to Transindividuation.* Abingdon, OX: Routledge, pp. 74–91.
Bazzano, M. (forthcoming) *The Affect Therapy Manifesto.* Oxford, OX: Mud Pie.
Boscovich, R. J. (2015) *Theory of Natural Philosophy*. London: Forgotten Books.
Deleuze, G. (1988) *Spinoza: A Practical Philosophy*, trans. Robert Hurley. San Francisco, CA: City Lights.
Geue, T. (2025) *Major Corrections: An Intellectual Biography of Sebastiano Timpanaro.* London: Verso.
Hinton, D. (2020) *China Root: Taoism, Ch'an, and Original Zen.* Boulder, CO: Shambala
Laplanche, J. (1988) *Essays on Otherness*. Abingdon, OX: Routledge.
Mikami, K. (2016) *The Body as Vessel: Approaching the Methodology of Hijikata Tatsumi's Ankoku Butoh*, trans. R van Hensbergen. Birchington, KNT: Osaru Books.
Nietzsche, F. (1978) *Beyond Good and Evil: Prelude to a Philosophy of the Future,* trans. R.J. Hollingdale. London: Penguin.
Nietzsche, F. (2001) *The Gay Science*. edited by Bernard Williams, trans. Josephine Nauckhoff. Cambridge, NY: Cambridge University Press.
Schaefer, D. (2016) *It's not what you think: Affect Theory and the power to take to the stage.* https://dukeupress.wordpress.com/2016/02/15/its-not-what-you-think-affect-theory-and-power-take-to-the-stage/ accessed 31 Dec. 25.
Spinoza, B. (1996) *Ethics*. edited and trans. by Edwin Curley. London: Penguin.
Waddell, N. & Abe, M. (Eds) (2002) *The Heart of Dōgen's Shōbōgenzō.* New York: New York University Press.
Weixin, Q. (1990) *The Sayings of Chingyuan Weixin*, trans. G. Terebes. Budapest: Officina Nova.

Chapter 2

Shake it off

Vicarious Trauma, referred pain and othered people

Zoë Krupka

Who was it that said the past is another country? It's not another country; you just don't live there anymore.

There was a day just this past year when I began to put an end to working as a psychotherapist. This possibility had been in my mind for at least two years, but it had taken me time to believe it, to trust that it could be both a real thought and an action that might begin to lead me out of the woods of my own loss of meaning and direction.

As you can see, and I can see writing this, I must have blamed my sense of painful wandering on my work. Something was amiss in what I was doing. Was I no longer suited to sitting with people in the dense effort of remaking a life? Was I tired, bored, lonely or beside myself with desire for other experiences or another self? Was I in some way wounded by my efforts? I do not have answers to these questions.

I spoke with people about this decision, friends, colleagues, my supervisor, the guy who cuts my hair and the vet who cares for my cats. If I was distilling some kind of thematic analysis of their responses and reflections, the headings would read something like this: people are complicated and difficult, people ask a lot of you, people's stories stick like grass seeds in your ears and people's pain becomes your pain and too heavy to carry. Their reassurances all clustered around the idea of my essential purity and separateness and the danger posed by the distress of the unnamed. I had become stained, marked by bruising stories and needed to retreat, to wash off the painful lives of others.

There is a sister process to this attempt to separate from the pain of other people. When I'm lying in bed at night woken by shame about a transgression and I turn it over and over, I often find it to be pedestrian, common for people like me. I tell myself that I don't get to see myself as a monster. How grandiose. Perhaps everyone is monstrous and filled with shadows? I mean to soothe my catastrophic anxiety in this way. And yet in my work to get back to sleep by convincing myself that this common act of ignorance or dismissal is as small as a new kangaroo, there is a part of me that knows that even these everyday hurtful acts could still be part of someone else's giant, compounded wound. And like a school of piranhas, these

DOI: 10.4324/9781003669906-3

clusters of painful events can quickly devour someone with their tiny, ferocious mouths. Making light of them under the lamp of my own assumed goodwill keeps me looking like Narcissus into the mirror of my own feelings.

I've swum with my own piranhas over the years, and I'm not saying for a minute that other peoples' pain hasn't hurt me. Of course it has. The man alone on his farm contemplating suicide with only an old dog for company. The woman who fled to this country only to encounter the slow violence of endless detention. There are so many people whose pain has taken up residence in my heart. I don't question that. What I do want to ask, is why shouldn't it? Why shouldn't the pain other people feel hurt me too?

I'm writing this chapter as more people are dying and displaced at the hands of ongoing colonial projects[1] than ever before and the disparity between rich and poor has never been greater. And for those of us working in the so-called helping professions, there has never been so much information on how to maintain our health and wellness, so many ways to stay clean in a dirty world. Self-care, a practice that began with the fight against racist medical discrimination (Ortiz, 2013), has been swallowed up by late stage white supremacist capitalism into a multi-billion-dollar industry that appears to be selling candles and services run on people smuggling to those who might be in danger of experiencing horror.

Even fascism is acceptable as long as it's in the service of hacking health. Someone I supervise who is struggling to manage their alcohol consumption has just sent me a text. In the app they use to support their semi sobriety, today's motivational quote is from Margaret Thatcher. *You may have to fight a battle more than once to win it.* I text back another quote from the woman who called Nelson Mandela a terrorist. *I am extraordinarily patient provided I get my own way.*

Within the macroclimate of public health in the white global north, there is a blossoming, invasive new language for caring for those with ongoing emotional and physiological distress. The words trauma-sensitive and trauma-informed practices are ubiquitous, but when we are workers trained to assist the traumatised, we are told to be mindful of *vicarious* trauma. The idea that trauma could be acquired vicariously began with the study of the impact of trauma work on trauma therapists and is defined by Caringi and Pearlman (2009) as "the negative transformation in the helper that results (across time) from empathic engagement with trauma survivors and their traumatic material, combined with a commitment or responsibility to help them" (pp. 202–203).

Somehow, like the belief in transference or self-actualisation, this idea has found its way into the vocabulary of most Eurocentric approaches to managing distress in other people. Like the still beloved concept of parallel process,[2] it has embedded within it the idea that the origin story for the replication of dysfunctional dynamics lies with the trauma survivor seeking help.

The myth of vicarious trauma goes something like this: you're meant to be very cautious with this trauma thing because it's apparently contagious and this is not as it should be. One person is really the sick one and the person who has contact with them, particularly if they're trying to be helpful, can become sick with their sickness and that's something that shouldn't happen. A natural and right membrane has been fractured and requires repair and bolstering. To facilitate this fortifying clean-up, the offending material must first be identified and separated out. And to do this requires new words that can hold the soil which has now become dirt.

The concept of vicarious trauma is an affective container that positions trauma as an object; isolated, quarantined and divorced from its birthplace. Trauma has come to be understood as a sort of feeling parcel that lives in the bodies of others and away from the collective and individual selves of the ongoing colonial project. You can catch it from someone who has been hurt, but the pain you feel can never be yours – it has nothing to do with you. When we speak of trauma as vicarious, it's as if the pain of witnessing harm is an accidental departure from an unconscious utopian expectation whose mirage is reinforced each time we name ongoing, distorting and inconvenient pain as an aberrant transmissible response.

In an interview about his hugely influential book on the psychophysiology of trauma, Bessel van der Kolk, physician and former President of the International Society for Traumatic Stress Studies, spoke to his companion about what trauma studies now have to offer the world:

> We're at the beginning of a new scientific epoch, he told me, of understanding the truth about trauma: Finally, humanity can hope to free itself from the cycles that have dragged us through eons of war, violence, and poverty. Someday soon, he told me, finally, we will all become clean.
>
> (Carr, 2023)

Reading this, I think of a student in one of the first classes I ever taught. It was a unit called grief, loss and trauma. Because of the Australian government's education policy at the time, a course in community services was subsidised for those who had fled here as refugees and asylum seekers. Why not train those in need of care to care for others? In my class were students from the former Yugoslavia, Sudan, the Democratic Republic of the Congo, Ethiopia and Eritrea and two white Australian students who were the first in their families to study past high school. I was a white Canadian middle-class pansexual migrant studying for my master's in counselling and psychotherapy. I had a small child, a dog, a job in a youth homelessness service and a house with a garden. The traumas of war lived with my father and were stories, fears, loves, aversions and felt senses to me. For most of my students, they were alive and ongoing.

This particular day we were speaking about grief. We had begun to cover trauma the week before. M, who had fled the Democratic Republic of the Congo and was not in class the previous week because she had been ill, raised her hand. Everyone raised their hands to speak no matter how many times I suggested we could all just talk when we had something to say. She asked, *What is it then, the feeling, when your children are killed in front of you?* A stillness came over me. I did not know what to say, so I was silent for a few seconds. Then R, whose sisters and father had been shot by their neighbours in Kosovo, answered her. *M, that's not grief, that's trauma. We did trauma last week.* M seemed satisfied with this answer and I had nothing to add. They had learned that their stories were large and could hurt others and our readings and the words in them helped to keep these stories in storage. We knew they were there, but we weren't allowed to feel them together. M never spoke of the killing of her children in class again. But eventually she did speak of the people they had been. We listened.

The title of Bessel van der Kolk's bestselling book is *The Body Keeps the Score: Brain, Mind and Body in the Healing of Trauma*. A total of 33, 330 Kindle readers have apparently highlighted the following passage of his work since its publication as an eBook: "For real change to take place, the body needs to learn that the danger has passed and to live in the reality of the present" (2015, p.24). This was the core of the thesis I was meant to pass on in that class of people whose current traumas were living and breathing, and whose past traumas would be with them till death and live on in those they loved and who had loved them.

And so on. The body is a scoreboard.

I am certain that some of the students in that room on that day we were speaking of grief and returning to trauma had experienced some of what van der Kolk would describe as *healing*. Their nervous systems may have settled, muscles softened and a capacity to think clearly and to live outside of the shadows of the recent past may at times have returned to them. There were days when there was so much hysterical laughter in class that the department head called me in to his office to tell me off. *What are you actually teaching?* He would ask me. I think now that we were laughing at the absurdity of this myth of healing. Of course, we can't return to our essential unsullied selves. We can't carve off the parts we don't like and we can't go back in time. But I think we all longed together for exactly that, and the poignancy of that longing made us giddy with dissonance.

What they were learning and what I was meant to teach them with this new language of trauma and recovery was that like bombs, their traumas could be deactivated, and that in this process, care needed to be taken not only to prevent internal re-explosion (re-traumatisation) but also the wounding of others who would bear witness to their pain. Trauma, we were learning, always needed to happen last week.

For those of us hearing the trauma tales of others, the concept of vicarious trauma builds on this fantasy expectation of a severed, bleached form of healing and essentially pathologises the necessary pain of bearing witness to unspeakable acts. It repositions us from witnesses to spectators. Now it is this other thing – vicarious trauma – that becomes the real danger to the helping professional, allowing worldly perpetrators – state-sanctioned violence and terror, poverty and countless individual acts of cruelty – to walk free. The affects imprisoned within the container of vicarious trauma can now be socially instrumentalised by naming not the impact of violence or those responsible, but instead labelling the telling of traumatic truths as potentially deadly and ongoingly contagious. The biopolitics of these illegal feelings now function like Ruby Hamad's (2019) description of white tears; as a narcissistic reversal of responsibility where the pain of bearing witness to trauma becomes more important than the pain of experiencing it.

We are taught to congratulate ourselves on our resilience working with the violated and rewarded for our capacity to prevent the sharing of pain with others in workplaces that are slowly becoming feeling laundering machines. This is part of why the act of offering a trigger warning is so fraught. Not because it is impossible to be prepared for distress, or because it's wrong to offer caution to those who may be raw, but because the belief in one's right to not be hurt by the pain of others is so deeply suspect.

The idea that the pain of traumatic events is meant to confine itself to one persons' body is wounding on an incalculable scale. This fencing of emotional territory is part of the colonial project, envisioning a time of complete healing that is a full integration of a person to the world-as-it-is, where the pains of the past only exist in the past and never in this present that could be safe and perfect. That is the neoliberal colonial dream, to come together as one, where former sovereignties and the ongoing violence of erasing them are forgotten and where things can be restored, reconciled and made whole again in a single unified nation. A scoreboard was erased.

In my cupboard, I have a fat fake fur coat. It's yellow, the colour of a cartoon baby chick. It's warm, and when I'm feeling in need of comfort and protection, if the weather is cold enough, I wear it.

The technology for fake fur has come a long way. More and more it feels like real animals, it is harder and harder to perceive the acrylic it's made from. Fake fur is a kind of affective vessel, no longer an imitation of a real dead animal killed to make a garment, but a thing in itself – an animal that was never alive. How it was sold to me was not simply its deeply satisfying tactility, but also through a kind of permission to adore a furriness that is inherently beautiful and kind because it involves no killing, advertises my anti-fur wearing goodness all while allowing me to walk in the cold and remain warm. I can poach the plasticised beauty of the real animal. The killing of animals for fashion and sport is still going on, masses of it. Fake fur has done nothing to change that. It is a symbol of change, a trauma-informed stand-in that provides an octopus ink cloud behind which more killing can hide. The blanket of fake fur in late-stage white supremacist capitalism is a miniscule part of a wider system of engulfment, where pain is rebranded into harmless artifice. The bad things are over and the good things are here, now, clean and soft as a baby bird.

The denial of our shared affective ecology embedded in the concept of vicarious trauma has made it a very sticky label in the colonial helping professions, particularly with people whose traumas are systemic, pervasive and ultimately preventable. Separateness, when it comes to the pain of others, is one of the foundations of settler societies and sits at the heart of how we learn to help in the white university. It's a terrible illusion that professional roles can control affective transmission. Of course, that's not possible. But what has been made possible is so much worse.

This transmission of affect now stands in for the original violence, a scapegoat that can be treated with conversion therapy, convinced that there is in fact no need to be drawn to the pain of others.

Preventing vicarious trauma is also meant to buffer the worker against burnout. But what for? To be able to go on working. The fable of vicarious trauma is also a neoliberal fable. It is a disease of the worker who can't go on. Hazmat suit pierced, they have moved from spectator to participant – changed teams from the living to the dying. They can no longer perform in the service of keeping traumas contained in the bodies of those who so often have been wounded by systems dependent on their suffering for survival, and again by the very systems they have been directed to for assistance.

Of course, there is affective resonance with the distress of others. When that hurt is projected in a discourse of othering, then it becomes a disease rather than an impact with a known source. I don't want to hold on to a twisted hope of redemption, understanding, healing or cure for a weasel illness. Why not be devastated? Who shouldn't be devastated? I am trying not to be ashamed of cynicism or despair when they descend upon me. There is no separation between me the worker and me the person. The very idea of this separation creates a fracturing, both social and internal, between not only the body and the mind but also between the individual and the world.

You may not have heard that perhaps right at this very moment, magpies across "Australia"[3] are messing with well-meaning university scientists who are out to study them. These black and white passerine birds are removing data trackers from each other's feathered bodies. They can't remove their own pesky stalking devices, but they can take them off each other. What have studies ever offered them?

When I first heard this story, I found myself moved to being hopeful about the prospect of people understanding more about the true intelligence and coolness of magpies because I find them especially awesome. To my Turtle Island-born ears, their songs sound like an underwater chorus and it lifts something inside my chest. They fiercely swoop my cats and kids on bicycles and remember the people that have wronged them for life. Despite what we've done and are still doing to birds, actual birds and the habitats we all depend on, they're still busy acting like their lives are their own, whether we're thinking about them or not – responding to the pain of others, feeling the pinch of the trackers on each other's backs.

To move out of vicarious trauma's fairy tale forest, where I have become lost searching for food that is not poisonous and won't put me to sleep for a thousand years, I find a need to move towards feelings of destruction – to settle into the impossibility of a safe environment; to feel sick, broken and in despair – not as some kind of rite of passage to the other, beautiful heaven side of cleanliness, healing and a well-stocked gut microbiome, but as a way to avoid a deadening and deadly disconnection; and to notice the desire for purity and to spoil it. When I can interrupt this habit of fantasising my separateness and yours through this policing of traumatic affect and instead accept that I am hurt by what hurts you and often a cause or a beneficiary of your pain, then the possibility of addressing the roots of trauma and traumatic events opens wider. Sickness becomes the window.

Eventually I left the university where I first taught grief, loss and trauma. The hours allocated for everything from course preparation to meetings with students, already so little, had been reduced by more than half. I was hopeless and lost. Not so different to where I am now. Sick and tired.

Sitting outside at the edge of the carpark on my last day I saw M. She came to sit beside me. She was finished her course and working in an organisation for bereaved parents. We said goodbye and she took my hands. *They are always with me, my dead children and now they are with you too.*

Notes

1 I'm thinking here of Evelyn Nakano Glenn's definition of settler colonialism - "A settler colonialism framework can encompass the specificities of racisms and sexisms affecting different racialized groups…while also highlighting structural and cultural factors that undergird and link these racisms and sexisms." – and projects are those current and ongoing wars over territory and control, both political and economic. Glenn (2015).

2 Parallel process, imagined originally in a psychoanalytic context by Searles (1955), was the idea that in supervision, the dynamics within the patient and then in the therapeutic dyad, could be replicated unconsciously in the supervision dyad. This distorting replication then potentially obscured the pathway to cure.

3 The practice of putting Australia in quotation marks is to highlight that this continent is a multitude of unceded First Nations lands.

References

Caringi, J., & Pearlman, L. (2009). Living and working self-reflectively to address vicarious trauma. In C. A. Courtois & J. D. Ford (Eds.). *Treating complex traumatic stress disorders: An evidence-based guide* (pp. 202–222). Guilford Press.

Carr, D. (2023, July 31). Tell me why it hurts: How Bessel van der Kolk's controversial theory of trauma became the dominant way we make sense of our lives. New York Magazine.

Glenn, E. N. (2015). Settler colonialism as structure: A framework for comparative studies of US race and gender formation. *Sociology of Race and Ethnicity*, *1*(1), 52–72.

Hamad, R. (2019). *White tears, brown scars: How white feminism betrays women of color.* Melbourne University Publishing.

Ortiz, K. (2013). *Body and soul: The Black Panther Party and the fight against medical discrimination.* University of Minnesota Press.

Searles, H. (1955). The informational value of the supervisor's emotional experiences. *Psychiatry*, 135–146. https://doi.org/10.1080/00332747.1955.11023001

Van der Kolk, B. A. (2014). *The body keeps the score: Brain, mind, and body in the healing of trauma.* Viking.

Chapter 3

Clients being beside themselves

Affect and ecstatic vulnerabilities in the therapy room

Konstantinos Tzikas

"What's the deal with these so-called 'femicides'? A handful of women, considerably fewer than men, mind you, get killed every year and suddenly there's such a fuss about it! They must have had it coming!". Fondas, a 41-year-old client of mine, would sometimes explode during our sessions, articulating remarks such as the above. More than once, he had stormed into my office, relating his difficulties: how he can no longer catcall a woman who wears what he considers provocative clothing; how he is attacked by what he believes are proponents of political correctness whenever he attempts to openly express his views, which to my ears are patently misogynistic, homophobic and racist; how climate change is a big sham; how aghast he was with a recent artwork by a female artist, a pink version of the Greek flag made out of bed sheets, serving as a monument to femicide victims in Greece.

Working with this client over the course of several months had been difficult. In my sessions with Fondas, whenever he turned to such ranting and raving, as I silently (and judgementally) labelled it, I would hold my breath, confronted with beliefs very different from my own. As a follower of person-centred therapy, I could feel the three necessary and sufficient conditions for therapy, as laid down by Carl Rogers (1957), being challenged: my congruence, empathy and unconditional positive regard towards this person would be momentarily shaken. What I had failed to register at the time was that I was caught in a circuit of *affect*, not unlike what was happening with other clients of mine, albeit this affect was unpleasant and unfamiliar. In a way, I was being incinerated by this affect, much as Fondas himself was. Bodies can absorb feelings as easily as fire: affect jumps from one body to another, stirring up tenderness, breeding shame, igniting rage, provoking fear (Gibbs, 2001).

Affect, of course, is a notoriously ill-defined concept, subject to multiple interpretations.[1] Arguably, much of its power derives from its opacity. I often return to the opening sentence of Teresa Brennan's seminal book *The Transmission of Affect* (2004) as it succinctly yet poetically encapsulates what affect is all about: "Is there anyone who has not, at least once, walked into a room and 'felt the atmosphere?'" (p. 1). Significantly, as she points out, "[t]he 'atmosphere' or the environment literally gets into the individual", as this transmission of affect can even

DOI: 10.4324/9781003669906-4

induce physical and biological changes from one body to the next. Haven't we all perhaps experienced some such changes, whether we have found ourselves amid a cheering crowd of football fans or as part of a protesting assembly in the streets or in any other occasion invoking a collective feeling? In all these cases, there is an *affective contagion* at work. The concept has been theorised by various thinkers over the centuries, from Spinoza and David Hume to Deleuze and Guattari to Silvan Tomkins and contemporary theorists such as Brian Massumi and Sara Ahmed. Their outlooks on affect may differ but they tend to agree on one point: affects are migratory and sticky. For instance, Félix Guattari (1996) has discussed "this transitivist character of affect" that "sticks to subjectivity" (p. 158), while Ahmed (2010) has playfully suggested that an affect "rather like Velcro, [...] tends to pick up whatever comes near" (p. 40). And theorists also concur on another point: unlike feelings or emotions in the conventional sense,[2] affects are not private or personal; they do not belong specifically to someone; they are not internal and then become externalised; rather, they move and flow. As social anthropologist Eirini Avramopoulou (2018) explains, glossing Ahmed, affects do things, namely "they connect and bind bodies to each other, mediate the relationship between the psychic and the social, the individual and the collective, and, without settling somewhere, at once create surfaces and set boundaries" (p. 30).

Doesn't this affective contagion, this leaping of affect from one body to another, also hold true during therapy? As therapists, haven't we sometimes felt our own breath changing when facing a client whose breathing is visibly difficult? Or our own eyes tearing up while confronted with a client's tears? Affects are unveiled to us in all their sticky glory as we sit there, *traversed* by them, as Deleuze and Guattari (1994) would put it. When Lone Bertelsen and Andrew Murphie (2010), expounding on Guattari, insist that affect "'sticks' to 'speaker' as much as the 'listener', it sticks in empathy and desire" (p. 155), they might as well be describing a typical therapy setting. Indeed, a therapy room is very much a scene where one of the participants walks in while the other one receives them, and both come to "feel the atmosphere" in the room, an image sharply contrasted to the popular conceptualisation of emotion as something internal getting "out".

However, Ahmed (2010) complicates the schema of affective contagion by making a crucial qualification: this transmission of affect is not merely a mechanistic process of affects jumping through bodies and invariably producing the expected results, given "[w]e might be affected differently by what gets passed around" (p. 39). What we perceive as an atmosphere, or something in this atmosphere, depends on our viewpoint or position within a space, of how we already enter and look at a space. In other words, "to be affected by another does not mean that an affect simply passes or 'leaps' from one body to another. The affect becomes an object *only given the contingency of how we are affected*" (p. 39, emphasis in original).

As therapists, we do have a viewpoint. How we view the atmosphere in the room and how we relate to our clients is contingent upon our angles, our *positionality*, i.e. the sociopolitical context and experiences that shape aspects of our identity such as gender, race, class, sexuality and ability status, the "disciplinary, emotional, and cognitive lenses that influence how we view the world" (Szanto & Strutt, 2022, p. 330). These lenses betray themselves in our contact with otherness. As David Takacs (2003) stresses in his study of the connection between positionality and epistemology: "Only by listening to others can I become aware of the conceptual shackles imposed by my own identity and experiences" (p. 29). Rogers (1951) has underscored how paramount it is for therapists to understand clients "from the internal frame of reference" of the clients themselves (p. 494) rather than an external frame of reference projected on them – but doesn't this phenomenological approach also presuppose that therapists get well-acquainted with their own frame of reference, its scope, advantages and limitations?

Perhaps, then, it is important, first and foremost, to address where each one of us stands in relation to the various structures of power. This is what Donna Haraway (1988) has come to call our *situated knowledge*: knowledge, not in the sense of an objective vantage point, a thing-in-itself untainted by any sociocultural influences, a pure scientific authority in the vein of the Enlightenment. Rather, knowledge that is informed by our values, our historical and cultural context, our very bodies; therefore, knowledge as an inevitably subjective, relative, fragmented body of practices and discourses, an incomplete and even contradictory epistemology. To explain this further, Haraway draws on the well-worn, masculine, transcendent metaphor of "vision equals power", only to subvert it by inserting a decidedly feminist spin on it: removed from dichotomies of objective versus relative, body versus mind, she proposes a form of necessarily partial, specific, embodied knowledge, which "allows us to become answerable for what we learn how to see" (p. 583). Along those lines, she poses questions such as "How to see", "Where to see from", "What limits to vision" and "What to see for" (p. 587). If one transposes the same question onto the therapy room and replaces the verb "see" with "listen", the implications for how we stand vis-à-vis our clients *while* also acknowledging our positionality, our blind spots, privileges and biases are obvious.

In bringing all of the above concepts to the table, I am also obliged to come to terms with my own situated knowledge. To further illustrate my point on positionality: For this paper, I draw on my background in counselling, social anthropology, feminist and queer theory, while also acknowledging my status as a middle-class, able-bodied, European, gay cis man. Of course, this kind of *positionality statement*, unloading one's various identities, though commonly used by researchers in social sciences, can still seem a bit redundant, reductive or even self-congratulatory. Yet I do it here deliberately to underpin the argument that we can never entirely escape our positionality, no less when we are practising therapy.[3] Several contemporary schools of therapy point to this anyway; long gone are the days of the therapist seen as an objective, neutral authority. Tellingly, Rogers (1967) has singled out the genuineness or congruence of the therapist as the most important condition for therapy[4] – and perhaps there is an analogy to be made between congruence and situated knowledge.

My positionality also involves my sociopolitical engagement with this world. For instance, I am allied with LGBTQI+ and feminist causes. Moreover, I follow the post-structuralist school of thought. In that sense, I am fiercely, staunchly anti-essentialist. I don't believe there is a true, original, authentic self which predates a social self. I believe we are, right from the outset, even as foetuses depicted on a sonogram, as Judith Butler (1993) provocatively posits, gendered, shaped and moulded as ongoing products of discursive practices. Furthermore, I don't see therapy as a guide to wellness. I don't see it as a neoliberal project of self-improvement, an incessant pursuit of well-being. In fact, I find it vital that psychotherapy intersects with post-structuralism, social anthropology, queer and feminist critical thinking in order to question preconceived notions of humanity and humanness – notions which only serve to enhance neoliberal tenets such as responsabilisation, occluding the role that social and political forces play in shaping and motivating each one of us. Manu Bazzano (2023) has rightly pointed out how a post-structuralist stance "has very rarely been part of the conversation within contemporary psychotherapy" (p. 134). The reason, of course, being that psychotherapy has been largely rooted in a humanistic tradition, which, even today, carries traces of beliefs in autonomy of self, body/mind binaries and so on. These beliefs persist nowadays in positivist figurations of therapy as a will-driven instrument towards growth ("If you genuinely want it, you can change").

In view of the above, during therapy, my own positionality will inform, in part, how I come to perceive the atmosphere in the room, the outside getting *in* and *through* each person, what each client invites in the room, infused with the affect of our times. By way of example, I will briefly refer to different cases of clients bringing the atmosphere in the room, conjuring what Hannah Arendt (1998) calls "the potential space of appearance between acting and speaking men" (p. 200), i.e. the *polis* materialising inside the therapy room: (1) A non-binary client of mine shared their experience of going to the Athens Pride, despite their social anxiety, and how they succeeded in convincing their father to accompany them. Ultimately, it was a moving yet also stressful experience for them, marking one of the few instances they were publicly representing themselves as a queer person. (2) A young bisexual woman remembered the first time she ever went dancing at a queer nightclub and her exhilaration as she drank in the affect of the space, describing it as "safe", "inclusive" and "erotic". (3) A gay client of mine told me how once, as a boy with a fluid gender expression, he broke into a spontaneous dance during a family celebration, only for his gesture to be met with mockery from his relatives. (4) A trans client recalled the affect in the kitchen of his family home, sitting through uncomfortable dinners as his hostile family insisted on referring to him by his deadname. (5) Another gay client of mine narrated his experience of once testifying in court against the uncle who had been sexually abusing him as a child. He was enveloped in the homophobic atmosphere of the courtroom, as the defence attempted to rattle him, shame him and discredit him.

Vulnerability was a key aspect in all the aforementioned experiences. During our sessions, I readily recognised it in both myself and my clients, having experienced it my entire life as a queer person. I almost reeled from listening to their stories of thrill, danger, rage, exposure, shame and liberation. Dave Mearns and Brian Thorne (2000) once hailed the therapist's vulnerability as an important aspect, "far removed from the male stereotype of the clear-thinking, decision-making activist who leads his team (or his family) along the road to achievement, success and material security" (p. 77). Indeed, in some schools of therapy, including person-centred, it is perfectly acceptable for therapists to allow themselves to be openly moved by their clients and even communicate this to them; an avowed admission of being *affected*. However, I also slowly came to think whether vulnerability bears upon our own accountability as therapists, in tandem with Haraway's notion of situated knowledge. Maybe we are answerable not only for how we have learnt to look at things, our angle into the atmosphere of the therapy room, but also for our vulnerabilities. It prompted me to wonder whether philosophical postulations on vulnerability could help us broaden our thinking with respect to therapy – a field of work that, if nothing else, is predicated on vulnerability.

Vulnerability, ecstasy and abjection in a therapeutic context

In recent years, I have become increasingly interested in Judith Butler's analysis of vulnerability, partly influenced by the work of philosopher Adriana Cavarero. The latter, in turn influenced by Arendt, has asserted that the self is constitutively exposed to the Other from its birth onwards: simply put, each one of us forms a self by virtue of being exposed to everyone else's gaze, to everyone else's narrative about us and our lives. The so-called uniqueness of personal identity emerges, then, as insubstantial, as having "a totally expositive and *relational*[5] character" (Cavarero, 2000, p. 20, emphasis added), given we are formed as subjects only in relation to others, what Cavarero refers to as "[e]xistence as exposure" (p. 19).

Butler further builds upon the twin pillars of exposure and relationality in their problematisation of vulnerability. Following Cavarero's hypothesis that "we are beings who are, of necessity, *exposed* to one another in our vulnerability and singularity" (Butler, 2005, p. 31, emphasis in original), Butler contends that "learning how best to handle—and to honour—this constant and necessary exposure" (pp. 31–32) is absolutely vital for our survival. An exposure which cannot help but be primarily felt in the body: "Vulnerability implicates us in what is beyond us yet part of us, constituting one central dimension of what might tentatively be called our embodiment" (Butler, 2015, p. 149). Butler reminds us that crucial as it may be to fight for our bodily autonomy, sexual self-determination and other such sociopolitical causes, our selves, and by extension, our bodies are never, in fact, entirely our own in the manner prescribed by Cartesian metaphysics, as "to be a body is to be given over to others" (2004b, p. 21). Violently refuting the idea of a solipsistic self means that "bodies are always in some sense outside themselves, exploring or navigating their environment" and "[i]f we can become lost in another, [...] that is because the body does not stay in its own place". (Butler, 2015, pp. 211–212).

As a way of framing their reflections on vulnerability and relationality, Butler has introduced a notion variously stylised as *ecstatic*, *ec-statik* or *ek-statik*. In common parlance, "ecstatic" is a word that evokes mystical connotations and perhaps cannot be completely divorced from them. However, taking after Heidegger, Butler resorts to "the original meaning of the term as it implies a standing outside of oneself" (Butler, 2004b, p. 258). Indeed, the word "ecstatic" comes from the Greek verb *ἐξίστημι*, meaning "to stand beside oneself, to stand apart, to be displaced, to give up possession of something". Using the etymology of the word as a starting point in their radical reading of Hegel's notion of *recognition*, i.e., the idea that we all acquire self-consciousness and become social beings through a mechanism of mutual acknowledgement, Butler (2004b) proffers "an ek-static notion of the self, one which is, of necessity, outside itself, not self-identical, differentiated from the start" (p. 148). Running counter to the humanist idea of the unitary, self-contained self, Butler discerns a fundamental relationship between self and Other, in which the self "finds itself ambiguously installed outside itself" (p. 150), "cast, always, outside oneself, Other to oneself" (p. 148), subject to a form of splitting from the outset. It is a relationship that always entails a partial loss of self and is thus fraught with risk.

Therefore, for Butler (2005), when we utter the word "I" we are already placing ourselves outside of ourselves; there is no final, definitive moment upon which a return to our self is permanently achieved. We are always *out there*, in a way. For the philosopher, this intrinsic vulnerability we all share, not just by being mortal and thus injurable beings but also by dint of being responsive and receptive to the world around us, is an integral aspect of this ecstatic subjectivation; it is what constitutes us as humans. Moreover, as a radical opening to otherness, vulnerability carries ethico-political implications for our existence. By composing our embodied presence in this world into which we are thrown, it structures us not only as human subjects but also as politically engaged entities. Managing our immanent vulnerability serves a powerful (per)formative function.

Yet, *ἐξίστημι* can also mean "to be astonished or distraught, to be beside oneself with awe or surprise", as in the mediopassive form of the verb in Modern Greek, *εξίσταμαι*. With that in mind, Butler (2004a) adds another, more explicitly political dimension in their definition of the ecstatic, as they focus on populations who are beside themselves in a different way, in addition to the vulnerability we all inherently share and that is necessary for us to exist:

> To be ec-static means, literally, to be outside oneself, and thus can have several meanings: to be transported beyond oneself by a passion, but also to be *beside oneself* with rage or grief. I think that if I can still address a "we", or include myself within its terms, I am speaking to those of us who are living in certain

> ways *beside ourselves,* whether in sexual passion, or emotional grief, or political rage.
>
> (p. 24, emphasis in original)

What does it mean for a trans woman to walk the city streets? Or a Black person to publicly march? Or a man with a disability to try to embark on a departing ship, only to be pushed to his death by a ship employee, as we found out in September 2023 when this horrific hate crime, the murder of 36-year-old Antonis Karyotis, took place at the Port of Piraeus? For Butler, there are certain bodies that cannot help but be "beside themselves" – both in the sense of being displaced in more ways than once as well as in the sense of being overcome with grief, frustration, political rage, fear, resentment and shame. For instance, in addition to the interdependency, we all share as sexual beings whose desire leaves us vulnerable to betrayal or disappointment, LGBTQI+ people also have to resort to regulatory norms for legal recognition of their desire in order to survive – paradoxically enough, those same norms which often leave them exposed to danger. Butler and Athena Athanasiou (2013) caution us that our constitutive self-dispossession as ecstatic subjectivities, that fact that we can be lost to ourselves, in mourning or in love, "moved by others in ways that disconcert, displace and dispossess us" (p. 4), should not be used as an ideological alibi to legitimise a different kind of dispossession: precarity; dispossession of land and wealth; exploitation; social traumatisation; exclusion on the basis of biopolitical racism. Dispossession as an immanent human condition should be distinct from dispossession as an essentialist tool meant to frame specific populations as inescapably vulnerable and dependent and thus subject to paternalistic politics of pseudo-care (Butler, 2015).

There is no question, of course, that, time and again, specific dispossessed populations have been regarded by society as dirt, as "matter out of place" (Douglas, 2001, p. 36), to use a famous quote by anthropologist Mary Douglas. They have become *abject*, to use another famous term by Julia Kristeva: much like blood, excrement, cadavers or any other "jettisoned object" that is "radically expelled" (1982, p. 2) because it disrupts the social reason and symbolic order, trans people, immigrants, the homeless, those with disabilities, to name but a few, are framed as the impure waste of the body politic, cast off to the fringes of society via a brutal process of *abjectification*, "the mode by which Others become shit" (Butler, 1999, p. 170). These populations are perennially exposed to a differential violence upon their appearance in the public space of the polis. What has all this got to do with therapy though?

There is a very tangible reality of ecstasy and abjection that can find its way into our practices. Being there for people who are beside themselves is part and parcel of the therapeutic process. It's safe to say most of us have had clients coming into our offices being beside themselves. For instance, I've had a client who was beside herself with grief over the end of her romantic relationship. Or I've had several young clients who were beside themselves with anger about climate disaster or sociopolitical developments in Greece. At the same time, specific populations, such as those Butler mentions, will carry a special kind of vulnerability in therapy. Every client who has suffered a form of differential violence will bring something "of the streets" (be it protests, gay bashing, sexual assaults) into the session. Clients come to therapy having been abjectified by institutions such as family, state, school and church, as well as being self-abjectified, i.e. internalising this abuse, turning themselves into "waste" – what in person-centred therapy one might call the client's *incongruence*, that gap between self-perception and actual experience which, once perceived, generates anxiety to the client (Rogers, 1957). It would perhaps be irresponsible to overlook experiences of abjection and how they come into play, how they can also, like gas, spread around the therapy room in sessions with clients. Experiences such as coming out or being outed, being bullied, being sexually assaulted, being bashed or harassed, being shamed, or even navigating the pleasures and perils of non-heteronormative kinships and sexualities, from sex cruising to polyamory, are not just self-contained events; there is always an open channel with a social psychic life, with the collective atmosphere of living a precarious life as a non-normative subject.

Our work will inevitably converse with the ethico-political. We don't practise therapy in a vacuum. We are not astronauts coming in from the vastness of outer space and being decontaminated before we proceed to the interior of the spaceship. And this is true of our clients. The public and the collective will always encroach upon us since the therapy room, for all its privacy and confidentiality, is also a locus haunted by the public space of appearance. The therapy, or, for that matter, supervision room neither is nor should it be a perfectly clean, disinfected space. As Zoë Krupka (2021) has indicated, a supervision that functions as a decontamination chamber for mental health workers who come in contact with a toxic affective contagiousness does a great disservice to the idea of affective relationality, as it denies the ongoing mutuality of all relationships. As therapists, we owe it to ourselves and to others to be affected. We are accountable not only to ourselves and our clients but also to the world at large at any given moment, if one approaches this from an existentialist, Sartrean point of view.

At the same time, universalising our clients and eschewing their specific vulnerabilities are not conducive to therapy. Speaking to our clients' difference – rather than *diversity*, that dreaded term co-opted and capitalised on by neoliberal forces – from a place of situated knowledge, acknowledging our positionality instead of hiding behind a façade of neutrality, may be more to the point. I once recoiled in disbelief when a colleague stated something along the lines of: "It doesn't matter to me if the client is man or woman, gay or straight; I see a human being there above all". How can we make an appeal to universalism when not even human rights are truly universal, as Talal Asad (2000) has demonstrated, despite attempts by the human rights discourse to convince us of the contrary? And the value of human life is not universal either, as we've seen far too often even in the Western world where certain populations are subjected to what Achille Mbembe

(2003) has termed *necropower*, being abandoned to their deaths, as in the case of pushbacks and Mediterranean shipwrecks.

That being said, I must clarify that I am not trying here to reduce everything to identity politics. I understand the pitfalls of identity politics, which I still think can be sporadically useful when used self-reflexively as political categories. But being a gay therapist, for instance, does not guarantee one has valuable insight into specific experiences or that one is immune to carrying internalised homophobia themselves. Mearns (2003) has a point when he argues that a person-centred therapist needs "not to be an 'expert' on the client group or work to work expertly with the client" (p. 51). Being knowledgeable about specific client groups and concerns is not a prerequisite for a person-centred therapist to work with these groups nor does it necessarily predict a better therapeutic outcome, i.e. that the therapist will help create a space for the client to better relate to their experiences.

Nevertheless, if any such knowledge exists, it may significantly help, and therapists should ideally keep up to date with different theories and developments, adjusting their practice accordingly to be more expansive. We can't be working with trans clients or straight women pressured into motherhood without developing some familiarity with concepts such as transphobia or heterosexism accordingly. Racism, sexism and other forms of systemic oppression and violence are integral to a client's experience and cannot be excluded from the therapy room. One can't help but wonder whether contemporary therapy has been propagating itself as a process largely above and beyond any limitations, sociocultural, political, or otherwise, between therapist and client, to the detriment of the therapeutic process. Be that as it may, I argue that the closer therapists are to the body of situated knowledge they carry, the more attentive they can be, in an intersectional manner, to the intricacies, ambiguities, contradictions and inconsistencies in both themselves and their clients as they are moved by each other during therapy. It is by giving their due attention to these aspects that therapists can more readily swim into affective currents with their clients when the latter bring forth parts of their experience. And maybe therapists can share their own experiences of oppression sparingly, if they have any therapeutic benefit: even Rogers warmed up to the idea of therapists making use of their own selves in therapy towards the end of his life (Baldwin, 1987). But it must also be said that this affective interplay may involve any number of lacunae, which therapists and clients may or may not be able to fill, as I will discuss in the next section.

An affective choreography of anger and fear

The type of affective transmission I described is much more smoothly traversed when working with a client who shares a similar worldview with ours and supports values close to our hearts. There, we can afford to empathise and be passionate with another person's passion (though this is not without its own set of disadvantages[6]). In therapeutic groups of gay men, where I serve as assistant facilitator to existential therapist Leo Kalovyrnas, an affect is often palpable in the air when members of the group connect with each other and infuse the room with a charged atmosphere that "does something", as Ahmed would say. It is an atmosphere replete with a rhizomatic network of affective affinities. But can this therapeutic attitude also lend itself to work with clients whose beliefs differ dramatically from ours? A case in point: can I be there as a gay therapist with feminist and anti-fascist views for Fondas, a cis straight man who angrily unleashes sexist, racist, homophobic comments? What is the affect in the room when I listen to him dismissing what I consider an issue of utmost importance such as femicides? How to accommodate "toxic masculinity", in lack of a better word, in such a context?

Fondas had come to me with a specific request: "I want to live". At age 41, he wanted to live life in his own terms and introduce more joy to it. He felt he had lost precious time, often bound by a sense of obligation and duty even towards family members he loathed. At the same time, social interactions with people were a source of inordinate discomfort for him. He sometimes lashed out at them when he felt they were wasting his time or acting foolishly. However, as our sessions progressed, I would find myself annoyed, against my better judgement, whenever he veered off from his existential anxieties into outbursts about the deteriorating condition of our society, frequently disparaging the social causes I believed in.

It soon became apparent that the gaps between us were quite pronounced due to our markedly different positionalities. On a couple of occasions, it took a lot out of me to remain in a therapeutic position opposite him, most notably when he revealed how exaggerated he finds all the femicide reports. In that case, while it was clear that I was not agreeing with him – my silence and even a few very brief responses signalled that, much to his chagrin – I also struggled to maintain Rogers' core conditions for therapy, i.e. unconditional positive regard, empathy and congruence. Is this goal even feasible? How to remain genuine, empathic and accepting in the face of such difference? Congruence, in particular, posed a major problem.

Eugene Gendlin (1963) has suggested that the congruent therapist "need not always appear in a good light, always understanding, wise, or strong" (p. 110). If being genuine entails that the therapist "is being himself, not denying himself", "openly has the feelings and attitudes that are flowing in him at the moment" and "is willing to experience transparently any persistent feelings that exist in the relationship and to let these be known to his client" (Rogers, 1966, p. 185), I had to contend with my own unpleasant feelings and determine whether to communicate them to my interlocutor. For a few seconds, I could feel my own anger seething inside me, as he was taking an explicit stance against the various causes I have been actively supporting. At the time, I had not made the distinction between the feelings I harboured, pertinent to my personal history, and the affect that was shared between the two of us. The atmosphere in the streets, the affect, was there all right, but in a startling way: I was reading the room and I did not particularly like what I was reading.

It took me a while to realise that, while with other clients I was partaking in the affect of street protests or the vulnerability of a queer person walking the streets, with Fondas I was partaking in a different affect, one I was less familiar with, but still one that circulates in the political and the social. One that pervades many households in Greece: a reactionary rage and frustration against things deemed threatening to one's national, religious and sexual identity. Social backlash is inevitable and its very presence attests to the power and momentum that movements such as feminism are having right now around the world. Still, backlash is a different kind of song, a different kind of ecstasy, a different way of being beside oneself than I was used to, although with Fondas I had to march to its beat. Brennan (2004) reminds us that "the transmission of affect means that we are not self-contained in terms of our energies. There is no secure distinction between the individual and the 'environment'" (p. 6). I was experiencing this lack of secure distinction first-hand.

Working with Fondas was tantamount to a perplexing affective choreography. For the picture he painted proved increasingly more complex: at the same time as he was revolting against the changing perceptions of this world, he was also struggling with the fact he could no longer yell at people or verbally abuse them without feeling bad about it or realising he is increasingly developing some sort of "empathy", as he explicitly said, which is making his life more difficult. He was standing there, by his own admission vulnerable in front of me, something he's never done with anybody, including his long-time partner. And while Fondas projected onto me the image of an authority who will listen to his problems and provide foolproof solutions, I was being as vulnerable as he was, grappling with my congruence, as a gay man who has received his fair share of bullying in the past, now sitting across from a man who is at times aggressively masculine.

Ahmed (2017) has introduced in her writings the so-called "sweaty concept", one that comes to emerge, as she says, "out of a description of a body that is not at home in the world":

> By this I mean description as angle or point of view: a description of how it feels not to be at home in the world, or a description of the world from the point of view of not being at home in it. Sweat is bodily; we might sweat more during more strenuous and muscular activity. A sweaty concept might come out of a bodily experience that is trying.
>
> (p. 13)

My sessions with Fondas were, in that sense, "sweaty" theory and praxis in the making. I have often felt not at home in the world. Fondas has also felt not at home in the world, though for different reasons, being raised in an unstable environment and experiencing abandonment at a very young age, leading him to rely on ironclad notions of "right" and "wrong", alongside a mistrust and intolerance of other people. Fondas came to me, in the therapy room, beside with anger. But it wasn't just anger that was passed back and forth between the two of us, akin to a ball. There was also fear. Ahmed (2014) cites an excerpt from Franz Fanon's *Black Skins, White Masks* to illustrate how affect works: a little white boy sees a Black man on the street shivering with cold. Imbued with stereotypical notions of Blackness and Black masculinity, the boy thinks the man is beside himself with anger, shuddering with rage. The white boy fears the Black man, while the Black man fears the white boy's fear as it could lead to his own downfall. Fear, experienced here as a sensation of pervasive cold, does not belong exclusively to either of them; rather, it produces bodies differentiated from each other on the basis of an affective economy of fear. Fear meant not as personal feeling but as pre-personal affect: "Fear involves relationships of proximity [...] Such proximity involves the repetition of stereotypes" (p. 63).

Indeed, I was guilty of stereotyping Fondas as another "angry straight man" revolting against hard-won social victories. Therapists often pay lip service to the notion of multiplicity of selves, what Mearns and Thorne (2000) have named, in person-centred terms, our "configurations". Yet the fact remains we have been raised in a Western culture: we may still be tempted to believe in the indivisibility of an integrated self instead of adhering to a poststructuralist idea of disjointed, fragmented, or jarring assemblages of selves. I was unable to discern at first that Fondas' furious trembling also contained a deep-seated fear of our world, a demolition of his once unshakeable beliefs about what is wrong and right. And I hadn't grasped that his fear had migrated in me, arousing my own fear at being face to face with an aggressive man. Our affective economy charted out a psychic landscape with borders that kept us at a distance.

Massumi (2002) has famously equated affect with intensity, an "unformed and unstructured" (p. 260) intensity that can be nonetheless analysed. As Fondas and I remained there, there was risk in our encounter, in the intensity of our affect. Dialectics are never entirely innocuous, effortless and bloodless, as Bazzano (2023) reminds us in his analysis of Hegel: "Encounter with otherness necessarily implies separation as well as *negation*" (p. 130, emphasis in original). It is only through this relinquishment of self that a transformation can perhaps be brought about, as "the self comes to be probably constituted through encounter with otherness" (Bazzano, 2023, p. 131). And that is perhaps what I had initially failed to realise in my relationship with Fondas. Operating under facile assumptions about him, I was ignoring the reverberations and ripples running through us, the ebb and flow of our affective movements. With my situated knowledge, I had not done justice to his complexity, encompassing not just his personal history but also his positionality as a subject in a world perpetually permeated by affective, pre-personal forces.

Our differences notwithstanding, as several months went by, Fondas and I maintained our therapeutic rapport even as he began to experience a profound crisis when one of his loved ones succumbed to a terminal illness. This experience was changing him in ways he could not yet foresee, as he told me. Seismic shifts seemed to be afoot, as his absolute beliefs seemed shakier than before, including his beliefs in an afterlife: what was the meaning of it all? He was being drawn into a new experience of beside one-selfness: grief. As Bazzano (2023) asserts, "[g]rief, sexual passion, and furious rebellion free up the space commandeered by the self", which "can then become inhabited by a more immediate experience of finitude, vulnerability and agency" (p. 124). As Fondas and I explored together his experience of grief, alongside his own preoccupations over whether he was grieving "properly" or "successfully", it became obvious it catalysed something in him, perhaps offering what Bazzano calls "the opportunity of learning that embodiment [...] is a social phenomenon" (p. 124), that, far from being individualistic, our "coming-into-beings are both social and contingent" (p. 132).

Our shared uncomfortableness gradually began to be replaced by an unexpected camaraderie. There were heartfelt exchanges of gratitude; there was room for our disagreements; occasionally, there was even something tender in our interaction. Overall, this led to a weekly encounter which accommodated our difference: "Appreciation of otherness is ecstatic: it implies being moved outside of oneself. This form of displacement is what a self is" (Bazzano, 2023, p. 131). Tempting as it may be, I am not suggesting here a "happy ending" for our complicated relationship. Rather, what I am trying to formulate is that Fondas and I, to borrow Butler and Athanasiou's (2011) words in their analysis of the performative in the political, were "moved and even surprised or disconcerted by that encounter with alterity" (p. 4). The great Audre Lorde (1984) has rhapsodised about *difference*, "that raw and powerful connection from which our personal power is forged" (p. 112). She reminds us that we all forget the promise and potential of difference because "we have *all* been programmed to respond to the human differences between us with fear and loathing" (p. 115, emphasis in original). Of course, Lorde was referring to individuals bound together by joint causes when she proposed the notion of difference as an enriching and dynamic force. But wasn't the whole point, after all, for Fondas and I to be able to start "relating across difference" (p. 123) in order to connect on a deeper level? That joint cause was there, all right: therapeutic for both of us, I suspect.

Conclusion: towards performativity in therapy?

Therapy is ecstatic: not in a quasi-mystical sense that would confer on the therapist a status of secular shaman moving between different planes, but in the sense of an experience, like love or poetry, that compels us to "go beyond ourselves and move ecstatically towards others" (Bazzano, 2023, p. 150). If one taps into Butler's idea of vulnerability as ecstatic relationality and attempts to transcribe it in a therapeutic context, a question tentatively emerges: how can one embrace vulnerability in therapy without either forgoing it in favour of an image of the therapist as the strong captain at the helm or giving in to an idea of a therapist whose own vulnerabilities take up too much space, impinging on the therapeutic process? Evidently, there is no clear answer to that. But politics could again point the way. For Butler (2011), the answer when it comes to the political is that bodies carry a performative power. Bodies are political inasmuch as they are also performative. It is through the performativity of bodies, through the way they interact, especially in the "gap" between embodied presences, wherein this potentiality can be transformed into a political tool; an affective plurality that is perhaps most glaring and palpable in activist protests and assemblies:

> For politics to take place, the body must appear. I appear to others, and they appear to me, which means that some space between us allows each to appear. We are not simply visual phenomena for each other – our voices must be registered, and so we must be heard; rather, who we are, bodily, is already a way of being "for" the other, appearing in ways that we cannot see, being a body for another in a way that I cannot be for myself, and so dispossessed, perspectivally, by our very sociality. I must appear to others in ways for which I cannot give an account, and in this way my body establishes a perspective that I cannot inhabit.
> (Butler, 2011)

By the same token, isn't the therapy room, like politics, also a space of appearance given it involves bodies appearing and being there *for* the other in ways and perspectives which cannot be fully accounted for? After all, the polis, for Arendt (1998), is not an entity strictly demarcated by physical and geographical designations but an endlessly moving community, "the organisation of the people as it arises out of acting and speaking together", "the space where I appear to others as others appear to me, where men exist not merely like other living or inanimate things but make their appearance explicitly" (pp. 198–199).

If we carry Butler's line of thinking over to therapy, should we put notions such as authenticity, either for therapists or clients, temporarily to rest? Perhaps what is more needed is to insert some performativity in the therapy room: entertaining the idea we are not immanent organisms as is sometimes espoused by contemporary psychotherapy, including person-centred; instead, we are dynamic processes, ever in flux, permeable, playful, moving and moved in a continuous flow of affective contagion. Mearns (2003) has discussed how therapists need to be *beside* their client, i.e. "as close to the experiencing of the client as possible" (p. 55) rather than "*on the side* of the client", that is supporting them in the sense of sharing the weight of their decisions. But arguably, there is another dimension to be added in this *beside*: how can I also stand *beside myself* as a therapist vis-à-vis my client – an affirmation of ecstatic relationality, a self-displacement that is in simultaneous dialogue with what is happening both inside the client and in the outside world.

Let us for a moment imagine therapy as a performative gesture: we sit there, bathed in affects in a manner that expressly invokes our embodied presences as well as our distances, physical and otherwise, our bodies as sounding boards of the music in the streets, the protests and the counterprotests alike. In effect, we are singing more than discussing, to echo the well-known person-centred saying that we have to listen to the music behind the clients' words. The analogy is on-point, since music is often marked out as one of the most potent ways of transmitting the intensity of affect: "In a lot of cases, the pleasure that individuals derive from music has less to do with the communication of meaning, and far more to do with the way that a particular piece of music 'moves' them" (Shouse, 2005). But sometimes even active listening will not suffice. What if we are not "hearing the right music behind the words to realise true empathy" (Barry, 2020) due to insurmountable gaps in communication?

Thankfully, the body is still there. Not merely "the body of biology, a body of organs" (Bazzano, 2023, p. 241) but the body as "dark, plural, traversed by a multiplicity of sounds and smells and textures and tongues" (Bazzano, 2023, p. 233), the Deleuzian body without organs, the Butlerian body that "does not stay in its own place" (Butler, 2015, p. 212), the Foucauldian utopian, incorporeal, incomprehensible, opaque body that "is always elsewhere. It is tied to all the elsewheres in the world" (Foucault, 2006, p. 233). Massumi (2002) pinpoints the two quintessential markers of the body: "It moves. It feels. In fact, it does both at the same time. It moves as it feels, and it feels itself moving" (p. 2). Therapy is an embodied process of feeling and being felt, moving and being moved. It is something both more and less than words, since language can never fully encompass what is being traversed during therapy. And affects will stick on us, whether we like it or not, so we might as well embrace the idea that affect is what moves the world, not money – what Massumi (2002) calls the "invisible glue that holds the world together" (p. 217). But maybe I needed a client such as Fondas for this realisation to fully sink in.

Notes

1 Manu Bazzano (2023) proposes the following concise definition of affect: "[T]he pre-verbal, impersonal flow of life's intensity and immediacy traversing living organisms. Hard to assimilate, it is habitually translated within subjective human experience as sadness, desire, joy, fear, ecstasy, anxiety and so on. It is rendered as emotion, feeling and sensation" (p. 231).

2 In his explication of affect, based on Massumi, Eric Shouse (2005) makes a useful distinction between feelings, emotions and affect: "Feelings are *personal* and *biographical*, emotions are *social*, and affects are *pre-personal*". Emotions are the display, feigned or genuine, of a personal feeling, but "[a]n affect is a non-conscious experience of intensity", which "cannot be fully realised in language", and is "always prior to and/or outside of consciousness", "the body's way of preparing itself for action in a given circumstance".

3 That is not to deny, of course, that our various identities are, by definition, unstable: we can never perfectly and completely embody or inhabit them, despite our repetitive attempts (and resistance) to do so, what Judith Butler (1993) calls, particularly with regard to gender norms, their *iterability*, a lifelong and never entirely successful process of performing for the "Big Other". But we cannot escape identity: in Althusserian terms, we have all been interpellated to varying degrees of success.

4 "Our experience has deeply reinforced and extended my own view that the person who is able *openly* to be himself at that moment, as he is at the deepest levels he is able to be is the effective therapist. Perhaps nothing else is of any importance" (p. 189, emphasis in original).

5 Relationality can be defined as "a view of the world that underlines how no person or thing exists in isolation, because existence necessarily means being 'in relationship'" (Wijngaarden, 2022, p. 412).

6 Mearns (2003) has made a convincing case that having unconditional positive regard for a client should be not confused with "liking" the client; in fact, too a strong similarity in values between client and therapist is not necessarily a good thing, as it can cause over-involvement with the client.

References

Ahmed, S. (2010). *The promise of happiness*. Duke University Press. https://doi.org/10.1215/9780822392781

Ahmed, S. (2014). *The cultural politics of emotion* (2nd ed.). Edinburgh University Press.

Ahmed, S. (2017). *Living a feminist life*. Duke University Press.

Arendt, H. (1998). *The human condition* (2nd ed.). University of Chicago Press.

Asad, T. (2000). What do human rights do? An anthropological enquiry. *Theory and Event, 4*(4). https://muse.jhu.edu/article/32601

Avramopoulou, E. (2018) Eisagogi. Politikes eggrafes tou syn-aisthimatos. [Introduction. Political inscriptions of affect]. In E. Avramopoulou (Ed.), *To syn-aisthima sto politiko. Ypokeimenikotites, exousies kai anisotites ston syngchrono kosmo* [The affect in the political. Subjectivities, powers and inequalities in the contemporary world] (pp. 11–67). Nisos.

Baldwin, M. (1987). Interview with Carl Rogers on the use of the self in therapy. *Journal of Psychotherapy & The Family, 3*(1), 45–52. https://doi.org/10.1300/J287v03n01_06

Barry, R. (2020). Investigating the necessity of prior cultural knowledge for person-centred counsellors working with multicultural clients. *The Irish Journal of Counselling and Psychotherapy, 20*(1), 10–14.

Bazzano, M. (2023). *Subversion and desire: Pathways to transindividuation*. Routledge.

Bertelsen, L., & Murphie, A. (2010). An ethics of everyday infinities and powers. Félix Guattari on affect and the refrain. In M. Gregg and G. J. Seigworth (Eds.), *The affect theory reader* (pp. 138–157). Duke University Press. https://doi.org/10.1215/9780822393047

Brennan, T. (2004). *The transmission of affect*. Cornell University Press.

Butler, J. (1993). *Bodies that matter: On the discursive limits of "sex"*. Routledge.

Butler, J. (1999). *Gender trouble: Feminism and the subversion of identity* (2nd ed.). Routledge.

Butler, J. (2004a). *Precarious life: The powers of mourning and violence*. Verso.

Butler, J. (2004b). *Undoing gender*. Routledge.

Butler, J. (2005). *Giving an account of oneself*. Fordham University Press.

Butler, J. (2011). Bodies in alliance and the politics of the street. https://transversal.at/transversal/1011/butler/en

Butler, J. (2015). *Notes toward a performative theory of assembly*. Harvard University Press.

Butler, J., & Athanasiou, A. (2013). *Dispossession: The performative in the political*. Polity Press.

Cavarero, A. (2000). *Relating narratives: Storytelling and selfhood*. Routledge.

Deleuze, G., & Guattari, F. (1994). *What is philosophy?* (H. Tomlinson & G. Burchell, Trans.) Columbia University Press. (Original work published 1991)

Douglas, M. (2001). *Purity and danger: An analysis of concepts of pollution and taboo* (4th ed.). Routledge.

Foucault, M. (2006). Utopian body. In C. A. Jones (Ed.), *Sensorium: Embodied experience, technology and contemporary art* (L. Allais with C. A. Jones & A. Davidson, Trans.) (pp. 229–234). MIT Press.

Gendlin, E. T. (1963). Subverbal communication and therapist expressivity: Trends in client-centred therapy with schizophrenics. *Journal of Existential Psychiatry, 4*(14), 105–120. https://focusing.org/gendlin/docs/gol_2129.html

Gibbs, A. (2001). Contagious feelings: Pauline Hanson and the epidemiology of affect. *The Australian Humanities Review*. https://www.lib.latrobe.edu.au/AHR/archive/Issue-September-2001/gibbs.html

Guattari, P.-F. (1996). Ritornellos and existential affects. In G. Genosko (Ed.), *The Guattari reader* (pp. 158–171). Blackwell.

Haraway, D. (1988). Situated knowledges: The science question in feminism and the privilege of partial perspective. *Feminist Studies*, *14*(3), 575–599. https://www.jstor.org/stable/3178066

Kristeva, J. (1982). *Powers of horror: An essay on abjection* (L. S. Roudiez, Trans.). Columbia University Press. (Original work published 1980)

Krupka, Z. (2021). Feeling heavy too: Thoughts on the concept of vicarious trauma. *Psychotherapy and Politics International*, *19*(1), 1–3. https://doi.org/10.1002/ppi.1559

Lorde, A. (1984). *Sister outsider: Essays and speeches*. Crossing Press.

Massumi, B. (2002) *Parables for the virtual: Movement, affect, sensation*. Duke University Press.

Mbembe, A. (2003). Necropolitics (L. Meintjes, Trans.). *Public Culture*, *15*(1), 12–40. https://doi.org/10.1215/08992363-15-1-11

Mearns, B. (2003). *Developing person-centred counselling*. Sage.

Mearns, B., & Thorne, D. (2000). *Person-centred therapy today: New frontiers in theory and practice*. Sage Publications.

Rogers, C. R. (1951). *Client-centred therapy: Its current practice, implications and theory*. Houghton Mifflin Company.

Rogers, C. R. (1957). The necessary and sufficient conditions of therapeutic personality change. *Journal of Consulting Psychology*, *21*(2), 95–103. https://doi.org/10.1037/h0045357

Rogers, C. R. (1966). Client-centred therapy. In S. Arieti (Ed.), *American handbook of psychiatry* (*Vol. 3*, pp. 183–200). Basic Books.

Rogers, C. R. (1967). Some learnings from a study of psychotherapy with schizophrenics. In C. R. Rogers & B. Stevens (Eds.), *Person to person: The problem of being human* (pp. 181–192). Real People Press.

Shouse, E. (2005). Feeling, emotion, affect. *M/C Journal*, *8*(6). https://doi.org/10.5204/mcj.2443

Szanto, D., & Strutt, C. (2022). Positionality. Wijngaarden, V. (2022). In P. Ballamingie & D. Szanto (Eds.), *Showing theory to know theory* (pp. 329–336). Showing Theory Press.

Takacs, D. (2003). How does your positionality bias your epistemology? *Thought & Action*, *27*, 27–38.

Wijngaarden, V. (2022). Relationality. In P. Ballamingie & D. Szanto (Eds.), Showing theory to know theory (pp. 412–418). Showing Theory Press.

Chapter 4

Adorno and Benjamin on affect, freedom, and the *promesse du bonheur*

Anastasios Gaitanidis

In the twilight of the empire of reason, where the grand narrative of Enlightenment culminated not in universal emancipation but in administered society and mechanised death, a profound question emerges: how might we speak of freedom? The philosophical journeys of Theodor Adorno and Walter Benjamin unfold within this fractured terrain – a topology of thought born from exile, rupture, and the shattering realisation that culture and barbarism are not antipodes but dialectical companions threading through Western civilisation's tendentious march. To write of freedom in the aftermath of this catastrophe is to fathom the deepest paradox of our historical situation: that the very instruments designed to secure human liberation – rational calculation, systematic organisation, technological mastery – have turned into their opposites, becoming the building blocks of domination itself. Here, in the shadow of Auschwitz and the spectre of total administration, Adorno and Benjamin chart a course between the rocks of indifferent despair and naïve optimism, in the effort to keep alive the few shards of hope that persist even in the darkest constellations of history.

Their critical theory thus emerges not as a nostalgic retreat from modernity's achievements, but as an archaeological excavation of modern reason's buried violence, a dialectic that refuses the false consolations of syntheses and metaphysical absolutes. The philosophical tradition has long harboured dreams of reconciliation – between subject and object, universal and particular, concept and matter – yet these dreams repeatedly turn into nightmares. What presents itself as philosophical synthesis often conceals violence: the merciless subsumption of particularity under universal concepts, the reduction of qualitative difference to quantitative exchange, and the subordination of nature's plenitude to instrumental reason's homogenising grasp (Jay, 1984, p. 65). Within this constellation of thought, affect emerges as the somatic remainder – that which persists beyond conceptual capture, the body's mute testimony against idealism's claim that reality is fundamentally rational.

In Adorno's philosophical analysis, the relationship between concept and object constitutes violence's primal scene. Traditional metaphysics, culminating in Hegelian idealism, posits identity between thought and being – the seductive notion that reality is fundamentally intelligible, that concept can fully capture its

DOI: 10.4324/9781003669906-5

object without remainder. Against this identificatory thinking, Adorno (1966) positions his negative dialectics as thought thinking against itself, a philosophy that would "use concepts to unseal the non-conceptual" (p. 5) without claiming mastery over what exceeds determination.

The non-identical – that which escapes conceptual capture – emerges simultaneously as philosophy's blind spot and its unredeemed promise. It manifests in those fissures where our conceptual apparatus falters, where we encounter the irreducible specificity of an object that overflows our categories. "The name of dialectics," Adorno (1966) writes,

> says no more, to begin with, than that objects do not go into their concepts without leaving a remainder, that they come to contradict the traditional norm of adequacy... It indicates the untruth of identity, the fact that the concept does not exhaust the thing conceived.
>
> (p. 5)

This remainder exists not as transcendent beyond but as immanent critique of the concept's totalising claim. It manifests as suffering, as the body's irreducible witness against the world as currently organised. Physical pain, in its brute facticity, constitutes a non-negotiable "No" that persists as affect – the somatic dimension of experience that troubles conceptual mastery. For Adorno, freedom begins in this gap between concept and object – not as positive liberty but as determinate negation of unfreedom. It emerges from recognising that our conceptual systems, economic structures, and social organisations systematically constrain human possibility.

The philosophical tradition's quest for systematic totality – from Plato's Forms to Hegel's Absolute Spirit – betrays an anxiety before the particular, a discomfort with what cannot be neatly categorised (Adorno, 1966, p. 12). This drive towards comprehensive systematisation reveals what Adorno diagnoses as the underlying fear that motivates traditional epistemology: the terror of confronting what remains irreducibly other, what escapes the net of universal concepts. The philosophical impulse to subsume all particularity under general laws, to reduce the manifold complexity of experience to manageable categories, emerges from an almost primordial dread of the uncontrolled and unpredictable. Yet this very attempt at mastery through conceptual domination paradoxically impoverishes thought, transforming the living multiplicity of experience into the dead uniformity of abstract relations.

However, the particular's resistance to conceptual categorisation – manifesting as the splinter in thought's eye – becomes not an obstacle to knowledge but its condition of possibility. The particular's stubborn refusal to be completely dissolved into universal concepts creates the productive tension that keeps thought alive and critical. It is precisely this excess, this surplus of meaning that spills beyond conceptual boundaries, that prevents philosophy from collapsing into mere tautology or self-satisfied system-building. Only where concept encounters its limit does genuine thinking begin. At these moments of breakdown, where the inadequacy of our categories becomes manifest, thought is compelled to acknowledge its own finitude and to remain open to what exceeds its grasp. This encounter with limitation does not represent failure but rather the real beginning of philosophical reflection – a thinking that remains faithful to the complexity of its objects rather than forcing them into preconceived moulds.

Walter Benjamin approaches this constellation through his concept of *non-sensuous similarities* – affinities between phenomena irreducible to logical identity or causal connection. These similarities manifest in the mimetic capacity that once allowed humans to recognise correspondences throughout nature. Modern rationality has attenuated this capacity, yet it persists in fragments – in children's play, in artistic creation, in those ephemeral moments when we experience the world not as dead matter to be manipulated but as a field of resonances and correspondences.

"Nature creates similarities," Benjamin (1933) writes,

> One need only think of mimicry. The highest capacity for producing similarities, however, is man's. His gift of seeing resemblances is nothing other than a rudiment of the powerful compulsion in former times to become and behave like something else.
>
> (p. 720)

This mimetic faculty represents a form of knowledge irreducible to conceptual classification, suggesting a relationship to the world preceding the subject-object split characteristic of instrumental reason.

Imagine the child who becomes the train or animal they imitate. This engagement with the other suggests a relation not through domination but mimetic transfiguration – through becoming-other rather than mastering the other. While appearing primitive from enlightenment rationality's perspective, Benjamin recognises in mimesis a critical potential – the persistence of knowledge that resists reduction to utility.

Language contains this mimetic element. Against viewing language as arbitrary sign system, Benjamin (1933) posits a "mimetic faculty" at its core – a capacity to recognise similarities exceeding mere convention. The onomatopoeic dimension of language, the gestural quality of certain expressions, and the bodily resonance of particular sounds: these aspects suggest language is not merely a representational tool but also a medium of embodied participation in reality.

The body emerges as crucial site in this dialectic – not the abstract body of biological science, reduced to mechanical processes, but the lived body of phenomenological experience, the seat of affect and sensation. For both thinkers, somatic experience registers what conceptual thought systematically excludes. The body remembers the violence enacted in progress's name; it carries civilisation's advancement scars.

This somatic memory constitutes a "sedimented history" (Adorno, 1951), the accumulation of experiences that shape our perceptual apparatus and affective responses. The body bears witness to what abstract thought forgets, to the suffering that remains the unacknowledged foundation of civilisation's achievements. It preserves a trace of what has been sacrificed in the name of progress, manifesting as the nagging discomfort that troubles our conceptual certainties.

"The body cannot be turned back into the envelope of the soul," Adorno (1951) writes in *Minima Moralia*, "but it becomes a sign of something that can yet be, a figure of hope. The less the body is submerged in the context of guilt, the more eloquently it stands for reconciliation" (p. 231). This passage suggests the body, when not entirely subsumed under civilisation's demands, becomes resistance and a locus for potential reconciliation. Somatic experience – affect in its immediacy – preserves a trace of what could be otherwise. The shudder before beauty, the visceral response to suffering, the embodied recognition of non-identity: these affective moments crack reified consciousness's smooth surface, momentarily suspending domination's compulsion.

Such moments do not themselves constitute freedom but create conditions for its possibility. They interrupt instrumental rationality's seamless functioning, creating spaces where alternatives might be glimpsed. This is why aesthetics occupies such a central place in Adorno's and Benjamin's philosophies. Art, at its most radical, preserves what instrumental reason excludes. It gives form to suffering without resolving it into conceptual clarity; it maintains the tension between universal and particular without forcing resolution.

The artwork's truth content emerges precisely from this tension – from its refusal to reconcile contradictions prematurely (Zuidervaart, 1991, p. 87). It retains elements that conceptual thought overlooks, while providing a form that facilitates intersubjective recognition. This form does not domesticate suffering but intensifies it, creating conditions for recognition of what exceeds conceptual capture. The aesthetic experience – that moment when we encounter artwork not as commodity but as challenge to our habitual perception – constitutes a microcosm of freedom, a fleeting glimpse of relational possibilities beyond oppression.

These glimpses remain necessarily fragmentary. Any attempt to integrate them into a positive vision of reconciliation would betray their critical potential, transforming what exceeds conceptual capture into another concept. This is why both Adorno and Benjamin resist articulating a positive vision of utopia. Freedom cannot be directly depicted without betraying itself – it can only be intimated through unfreedom's determinate negation, through attention to what troubles our conceptual apparatus.

Both Adorno and Benjamin inherit from Jewish theological tradition a profound suspicion of direct representation of the absolute. The biblical prohibition against images (*Bilderverbot*) becomes, in their work, a methodological principle: freedom cannot be positively depicted without betraying itself (Adorno, 1966, p. 207). Any attempt to portray reconciliation directly would reinscribe identity thinking's violence, subordinating freedom's open-ended possibility to a determinate image which inevitably falls short.

This prohibition does not mean abandoning hope for reconciliation but maintaining it as negative image – defined by what it is not rather than what it is. Progress and catastrophe are dialectically entangled; freedom's unfolding remains inseparable from unfreedom's history. This insight transcends mere pessimism. It recognises that only through confronting historical development's catastrophic aspects can we discern the fragile possibility of another way of being.

The *promesse du bonheur* arises from this tension, not as a guaranteed future state but as a possibility suggested through the determinate negation of existing conditions (Adorno, 1970, p. 136). It manifests in those moments when the non-identical asserts itself against conceptual capture, when affect disrupts instrumental reason's smooth functioning, when particular experiences resist subsumption under universal categories.

For Benjamin, such moments possess a messianic quality – they rupture the homogeneous flow of time, forming constellations where past and present interact critically. His concept of the "dialectical image" refers to these instances when historical understanding emerges in a constellation of tension. Benjamin (1940) suggests that,

> The past can be seized only as an image which flashes up at the instant when it can be recognised and is never seen again... For every image of the past that is not recognised by the present as one of its own concerns threatens to disappear irretrievably.
>
> (p. 391)

These dialectical images do not constitute historical knowledge in the conventional sense – they are not facts to be catalogued or events to be integrated into a continuous narrative. They represent moments when the past suddenly becomes legible in relation to present concerns, when what has been excluded from historical narrative suddenly asserts its relevance. Such moments possess a peculiar temporality – they are neither present nor past but what Benjamin terms "now-time" (*Jetztzeit*), a time charged with revolutionary possibility (Benjamin, 1940, p. 395).

This conception challenges progressive history narratives that see the past as inevitably leading to the present. Instead, it suggests history is composed of ruptures and discontinuities, of moments when what has been excluded from dominant narratives suddenly becomes visible. These ruptures possess political potential – they reveal the present arrangements as contingent, suggesting that what exists could be otherwise.

The critique of identity thinking extends to the subject itself. The unitary self – the "I" standing against the world as its master – represents a congealed form of domination. This sovereign subject, constituted through internal nature's repression and external nature's domination, is both agent and victim of reification. In *Dialectic of Enlightenment*, Adorno and Horkheimer (1944) trace how the unified self's constitution – exemplified by Odysseus binding himself to hear the Sirens – depends on inner and outer nature's domination (pp. 43–46). The formation of the rational subject requires the suppression of mimetic impulses, body disciplining, and affect's subjugation to cognitive control – mirroring society's domination of external nature through instrumental reason.

The subject's emancipation, paradoxically, requires this sovereign self's transformation – not its dissolution into undifferentiated nature but its opening to what exceeds its control. It requires recognising that autonomy emerges not through mastery but through responsiveness to what lies beyond the subject's constructive activity. This responsiveness is not mere passivity but active receptivity – an engagement with the world that neither imposes predetermined categories nor surrenders to immersion.

This conception resonates with Benjamin's notion of experience (*Erfahrung*) opposed to mere lived experience (*Erlebnis*). *Erfahrung* represents an engagement with sensuous particularity without reducing it to abstract categories (Benjamin, 1939, pp. 316–320). It suggests that cognition should remain receptive to what exceeds conceptual determination – to experience's affective dimension systematically excluded by instrumental reason.

The distinction between *Erfahrung* and *Erlebnis* captures modernity's paradox – the proliferation of stimuli accompanied by experience's impoverishment. Modern subjects are bombarded with impressions that remain external, failing to integrate them into meaningful narratives. This fragmentation of experience reflects broader social fragmentation: the division of labour that separates individuals from production's totality, the commodification that reduces objects to exchange value, and the bureaucratic rationality that treats humans as administrative units.

Genuine experience (*Erfahrung*) would involve reassembling these fragments – not through conceptual synthesis that imposes unity from above but through constellations that preserve particularity while revealing connections. Such experience would be simultaneously individual and collective, particular and universal. It would reflect the self's embeddedness in social and historical context without reducing individuality to a mere instance of a general category.

These implications extend beyond philosophical critique to psychotherapeutic practice. Just as negative dialectics maintains tension between concept and object without forcing reconciliation, a psychotherapeutic approach informed by these insights would remain attentive to what exceeds narrative coherence – to affective remainders troubling our meaning-making attempts.

In therapy's silent rooms where suffering seeks articulation, negative dialectics suggests a practice which witnesses the non-identical within psychic life – those fragments of experience resisting subsumption under diagnostic categories or therapeutic narratives. Think about the individual arriving bearing wounds exceeding linguistic capture – somatic symptoms, diffuse anxiety, and nameless dread. Conventional approaches might rush to translate these into recognised disorders, subsuming them under explanatory frameworks promising mastery through understanding. The negative dialectical approach instead remains faithful to suffering's materiality, attending to these symptoms as embodied critiques of existing conditions.

More precisely, this approach recognises that suffering is not simply a product of individual pathology but a fundamentally social response to a damaged and alienating social totality. It pays close attention to the ways in which individual symptoms are registering deeper social contradictions – showing how the human body testifies to what collective consciousness systematically represses or denies. The therapeutic task, then, is not simply reducing individual suffering using conventional treatments, but creating conditions under which it can be voiced or articulated as social complaint, recognisable as such and demanding response: an opening out to the complex ways in which personal pain or psychological symptomatology reflect broader structural distortions and systemic contradictions within society itself.

"The splinter in your eye is the best magnifying glass," Adorno writes (1951, p. 153). The therapeutic stance implied refuses to remove this splinter prematurely for comfort's sake. Instead, it magnifies the particular in all its discomfort, recognising that healing emerges not through suffering's transcendence but its transfiguration – through cultivating a relationship to pain which neither denies nor fetishises it.

Here is a fragment from an interaction with a patient that serves to demonstrate this therapeutic stance:

Elena shows up carrying what she refers to as "the weight of unnamed things" – a term that slips easily out of her mouth, like that of a prayer searching for its deity. In a hesitant manner, she talks about anxiety that precedes conscious recognition, and her unexpected, unbidden tears that cut across the smooth professional story that she has woven over her years as a company strategist. Her body, she is saying, is no longer her own – it has turned against her with tremors during presentations, with a racing heart at moments of actual stillness, with a persistent fatigue that no doctor's visit can explain.

"I feel like I'm living someone else's life," she confides, her voice heavy with the power of the non-identical affect asserting itself against the violence of the symbolic order. Her successful, well-calculated career has turned into a cage of market logic; each received promotion is a step further away from something she cannot name, yet feels as a nagging pain.

The space of therapy is becoming a dialectical laboratory as we engage with that which is more than her effort towards self-control. Her symptoms do not quite fit the familiar diagnostic categories; they are instead structurally akin to resonances between her physical pain and the dissolute disfiguration of contemporary life. The anxiety she suffers from is not simply personal pathology but her body's mute protest against the reduction of human possibility to exchange value.

On one occasion, Elena recounts a recurring dream in which she enters an infinite corridor of interchangeable doors, all leading to the same impersonal office. "I wake up struggling for breath," she says as her hand in involuntary motion goes to her throat – a movement that seems to speak before speech, conveying what she has not yet been able to say in words. This dream-image crystallises as a dialectical constellation where past and present collide in a moment of critical recognition.

The therapeutic work does not attempt to alleviate her pain so much as transfigure it by approaching her symptoms as a lens through which to see whatever was systematically excluded from her self-understanding. This process is an archaeology of buried potentials, caring for (and caring after) those moments when her petrified self-conception slips and slides away from her, when the gaps appear that reveal places where other ways of existing might be glimpsed.

And these tears, arriving without obvious provocation, are less events to be overcome than an articulation of the somatic gift that predates rational reflection and enables critical thought to begin. The healing that follows is not a cure for the disruption of seamless function, but a kind of growing of the ability to bear witness to what eludes conceptual capture. Elena starts to understand the symptoms she has been experiencing no longer as failures to adapt, but as resistances, and her body's refusal to be conscripted into the entirety of the machinery of capitalist neoliberal life.

In this way, the *promesse du bonheur* presents itself as an insight that flickers into life every time the non-identical shatters the glazed facade of reified consciousness, opening cracks within in which freedom might every so cautiously be breathed.

Such an approach transforms the therapeutic encounter itself. Rather than positioning the clinician as master interpreter rendering the unconscious conscious, it suggests a dialectical relationship where both participants engage in shared attention practice to what exceeds articulable understanding. The therapist becomes less expert knowledge possessor than companion in the negative, in the careful dismantling of reified self-understanding making space for what has been excluded.

This therapeutic stance resonates with Benjamin's (1940) conception of memory as active process – not passive retrieval of stored information but construction that transforms both remembered content and remembering subject. Memory work involves not merely recalling past events but creating constellations where they become newly legible in relation to present concerns. It involves attention to what has been excluded from dominant narratives – to experience fragments that trouble coherent identity narratives.

Memory work has also a political dimension that challenges progressive history narratives by highlighting breaks and discontinuities (Benjamin, 1940, p. 395). This examination of historical events sheds light on the gaps and shifts that challenge a linear progression of history.

Affect, on the other hand, intertwines with memory work by bridging the somatic dimension of experience and challenging the mind-body dualism. While it retains a connection to materiality that idealism often overlooks, it also plays a crucial role in how these historical breaks are perceived and felt.

This materiality is not positivist science's dead matter but vitality exceeding conceptual capture. It manifests when the body responds in ways our cognitive processing cannot fully account for – the tears that emerge without clear cause, the anxiety that precedes cognitive recognition of danger, and the spontaneous joy that interrupts melancholic reflection. In these involuntary reactions, the body remembers what instrumental reason forgets: the possibility of relation without domination, of recognition without subsumption. Such moments indicate a type of freedom characterised by receptivity to what lies beyond the individual self's boundaries, allowing for an engagement with otherness that occurs without appropriation.

Affect thus occupies a paradoxical position in the Dialectic of Enlightenment. It is both what must be disciplined in the formation of the rational subject and what persists as critique of that formation. The sovereign individual emerges through rigorous control of emotional life, through the subordination of somatic impulse to cognitive mastery. Yet in the very intensity of this control, affect reasserts itself as excess – as what cannot be fully integrated into the project of self-mastery.

Benjamin (1935) approaches this excess through his concept of "innervation" – bodily incorporation of external stimuli bypassing cognitive processing. In his photography and film writings, he explores how modern media technologies transform our sensory apparatus, creating possibilities for new perception forms and collective experience (Benjamin, 1935, pp. 117–118). These technologies, products of instrumental rationality dominating nature, nonetheless contain potential for mimetic world engagement – for forms of reception exceeding mere consumption.

This ambivalence captures modern experience's dialectical character – how the same forces producing alienation also create conditions for new relational potentials to emerge. Modern technologies simultaneously extend instrumentalisation and create possibilities for new perceptual forms – for collective experiential modes irreducible to individual consumption. Film, for instance, introduces an optical unconscious – revealing aspects of reality invisible to the naked eye and creating conditions for collective reception that transcends the bourgeois individualism characterising traditional art reception (Benjamin, 1935/2003, p. 104).

Both thinkers recognise affect as simultaneously the site of vulnerability and resistance. It renders us susceptible to the manipulation of the culture industry – mass-produced entertainment systematically adapting consumers to existing conditions – which exploits our mimetic capacities for commercial purposes (Adorno & Horkheimer, 1944, p. 31). It provides a simulated experience with standardised emotions that reinforce existing perceptual patterns instead of challenging them. Yet even within these degraded forms, traces persist of what exceeds instrumentalisation – moments when standardised narratives falter, revealing gaps where alternative possibilities might be glimpsed.

Freedom, in this framework, is not metaphysical absolute but historical possibility glimpsed in damaged life's gaps. It emerges not through the transcendence of material conditions but their transformation, occurring simultaneously in socio-economic structures and consciousness modes.

The notion of freedom cannot be encapsulated by abstract principles or universal norms. It emerges in specific instances of resistance to domination, in practices that foster receptivity to elements beyond conceptual capture, and in relational forms that do not involve subjugation. This involves careful attention to minute particulars where universal violence becomes evident and alternatives may be identified.

Such attentiveness necessitates a perceptual approach that uncovers the extraordinary within the everyday – what Benjamin (1929) refers to as "profane illumination" (p. 209). This pertains to moments when habitual perception is disrupted, the familiar suddenly appears unfamiliar, and what has been taken for granted reveals its contingency. These moments encompass both cognitive and affective dimensions; they involve not only intellectual recognition but also an embodied response that precedes conceptual articulation.

This mode of attention fosters an adherence to the specific characteristics of an object, rather than applying predefined categories. It accentuates the uniqueness of the non-identical, allowing for the recognition of elements that have been excluded from predominant narratives.

Such an approach suggests an ethics grounded in responsiveness to suffering and in recognition of non-identity between concept and object, between norm and case. This ethics would not seek to subsume particular ethical concerns under universal rules but would remain attentive to what exceeds such subsumption.

The ethical stance implied is not relativism but recognition that universal norms always fall short of particular cases they seek to govern – that ethics requires responsiveness to specificities exceeding rule application. It involves what Adorno (1966) terms "the addendum" (*das Hinzutretende*), a somatic impulse preceding rational deliberation yet not reducible to mere instinct (p. 229). This impulse constitutes moral action's material foundation, the bodily response to suffering that precedes ethical principles, yet makes them more than formal abstractions.

The *promesse du bonheur* remains in these interstices – not as a distant utopia but as an immanent critique, reflecting the possibility observed in instances where the body retains memories that concepts overlook. This promise endures as an approach that is loyal to particularity, while recognising patterns without confining them to rigid frameworks.

In our current era, technological rationality permeates every aspect of life, and the culture industry integrates critique into its promotional mechanisms, making the promise of happiness seem increasingly elusive. However, the intensity of domination leads to its own contradictions, creating areas where the non-identical resists conceptual constraints.

These contradictions manifest in specific points where the system generates resistance to its own functioning. They emerge not from outside the system but from within its own logic – from tensions between what the system promises and what it delivers, between formal equality and substantive inequality, between technological potential and its realisation under existing social relations.

The task involves discerning contradictions within the system and intensifying them – not through external critique that imposes abstract ideals but through immanent critique that reveals the system's failures by its own standards. This critique occurs not through judgement from an external perspective but through attention to what the system excludes yet relies on, such as the suffering that forms society's unacknowledged foundation.

Adorno (1951) writes in the final lines of *Minima Moralia*,

> The only philosophy which can be responsibly practiced in face of despair is the attempt to contemplate all things as they would present themselves from the standpoint of redemption... Perspectives must be fashioned that displace and

> estrange the world, reveal it to be, with its rifts and crevices, as indigent and distorted as it will appear one day in the messianic light.
>
> (p. 247)

This passage elucidates the paradoxical nature of Adorno's and Benjamin's philosophical projects – philosophy progressing through unwavering, relentless critique while upholding fidelity to the prospect of transformation. The "messianic light" they reference is not a theological certainty but a critical perspective that reveals the present as incomplete, laden with unrealised possibilities.

The standpoint of redemption they propose is not attainable in a positive sense – it cannot be assumed as a stable position. It only manifests fleetingly in instances where what has been accepted without question exposes its contingency. Nevertheless, their work encourages us to avoid both despair and naive optimism. It suggests that freedom emerges from recognising elements that transcend habitual perception and conceptual understanding, drawing attention to the somatic dimension of experience that underscores possibilities not currently realised by society's existing structure.

Adopting a genuinely critical attitude entails remaining open to those aspects of experience which continually elude conceptual capture and systematic classification, while providing a relatively robust basis for intersubjective recognition. Of course, this dialectical relation only serves to accentuate, rather than neutralise or displace, the non-identical elements that emerge within social relations, thereby creating space for those aspects of lived reality that have been systematically omitted from, or actively suppressed by, dominant discursive formations and hegemonic modes of understanding

This perspective can be described as a form of "negative utopianism," an orientation that finds the possibilities of transformative politics in the ongoing enactment of immanent critique rather than in any concrete positive vision or programmatic plan. Such a stance suggests that utopia fundamentally cannot be depicted directly or represented positively without inevitably losing its essential character as radical alterity, since any attempt at direct representation would necessarily reinforce the inherent conceptual violence and reductive tendencies of identity thinking. As such, utopia can only be thought of dialectically in terms of negation – by what it categorically is not and what it refuses to become – rather than through any positive catalogue of its assumed characteristics or concrete institutional arrangements.

In this respect, the *promesse du bonheur* persists not as a distant utopia but as a persistent critical outlook towards everything that currently exists. It appears as differential elements challenging conventional thinking, as affects exceeding cognitive control, and as particulars resisting integration into universal concepts. This potential arises when instrumental reason's efficiency fails, and we encounter elements that cannot be reduced to exchange value or conceptual equivalence.

This is the freedom Adorno and Benjamin intimate – not as metaphysical absolute but as historical possibility glimpsed in damaged life's interstices. Freedom that cannot be directly depicted without betraying itself, that can only be approached through unfreedom's determinate negation. It is sustained not by positive images but by relentless critique of what constrains human possibility – by loyalty to suffering refusing premature consolation.

As we attempt to come to terms with our own fractured landscape, where technology promises connection while deepening isolation, where abundance coexists with deprivation, where knowledge proliferates alongside profound disorientation, their negative dialectics offers not answers but a form of practice. It suggests an engagement with reality and a practice that neither surrenders to limitations nor pretends to transcend them, proceeding through immanent critique while maintaining openness to what exceeds society's present configuration.

This practice requires what Benjamin (1940) terms "weak messianic power" – the transformative ability to redeem those elements systematically excluded from dominant historical narratives and to activate the unrealised emancipatory potential that lies dormant in the past (Benjamin, 1940, p. 390). It involves the disciplined concentration on that which has been lost or annihilated in the name of progress and acknowledging the alternative horizons of possibility that have been foreclosed by specific historical trajectories. This is no mere nostalgia or romantic longing for a world that is lost, but an exacting form of critical engagement, which attunes itself closely to the present and recognises the possibility that the current social conditions could indeed be fundamentally different.

The project of negative dialectics by necessity remains inherently unfinished. Completing it would undermine its critical nature, turning an open-ended possibility into a rigid doctrine. Instead, it continues as an ongoing cultivation of thought and experiential modes that maintain openness to what lies beyond conceptual determination. It endures as a "promise" that can neither be explicitly articulated nor abandoned, sustaining itself through the relentless critique of unfreedom and careful attention to what instrumental rationality systematically excludes.

In this persistence lies radical hope – not in achieving a future state of perfection but in continuously transforming the present through a commitment to unrealised possibilities. This is the legacy offered by Adorno and Benjamin: a critique that avoids both resignation and false comfort, preserving the tension between what exists and what could exist without resolving into abstract certainty. This inheritance is received as a challenge rather than a dogma – to think critically against conventional thinking, to use concepts to unveil the non-conceptual, and to hint at freedom through the determinate negation of unfreedom. By accepting this challenge, we actively engage in the ongoing project of human emancipation, inspired by the *promesse du bonheur* that animates their work – not as passive recipients, but as active contributors.

Bibliography

Adorno, T. W. (1951). *Minima Moralia: Reflections from Damaged Life* (E. F. N. Jephcott, Trans.). Verso, 2005.

Adorno, T. W. (1966). *Negative Dialectics* (E. B. Ashton, Trans.). Continuum, 1973.

Adorno, T. W. (1970). *Aesthetic Theory* (R. Hullot-Kentor, Trans.). University of Minnesota Press, 1997.
Adorno, T. W., & Horkheimer, M. (1944). *Dialectic of Enlightenment: Philosophical Fragments* (E. Jephcott, Trans.). Stanford University Press, 2002.
Benjamin, W. (1929). "Surrealism: The Last Snapshot of the European Intelligentsia." In *Selected Writings, Volume 2: 1927–1934* (R. Livingstone et al., Trans., M. W. Jennings, H. Eiland, & G. Smith, Eds.), pp. 207–221. Harvard University Press, 1999.
Benjamin, W. (1933). "On the Mimetic Faculty." In *Selected Writings, Volume 2: 1927–1934* (R. Livingstone et al., Trans., M. W. Jennings, H. Eiland, & G. Smith, Eds.), pp. 720–722. Harvard University Press, 1999.
Benjamin, W. (1935). "The Work of Art in the Age of Its Technological Reproducibility." (Second Version). In *Selected Writings, Volume 3: 1935–1938* (E. Jephcott et al., Trans., H. Eiland & M. W. Jennings, Eds.), pp. 101–133. Harvard University Press, 2003.
Benjamin, W. (1939). "On Some Motifs in Baudelaire." In *Selected Writings, Volume 4: 1938–1940* (E. Jephcott et al., Trans., H. Eiland & M. W. Jennings, Eds.), pp. 313–355. Harvard University Press, 2003.
Benjamin, W. (1940). "On the Concept of History." In *Selected Writings, Volume 4: 1938–1940* (E. Jephcott et al., Trans., H. Eiland & M. W. Jennings, Eds.), pp. 389–400. Harvard University Press, 2003.
Buck-Morss, S. (1992). "Aesthetics and Anaesthetics: Walter Benjamin's Artwork Essay Reconsidered." *October*, 62, 3–41.
Jay, M. (1984). *Adorno*. Harvard University Press.
Zuidervaart, L. (1991). *Adorno's Aesthetic Theory: The Redemption of Illusion*. MIT Press.

Chapter 5

Making love to your data

On affect and post-qualitative research

Manu Bazzano

Introduction

From the 1990s onwards, the social sciences have witnessed the gradual emergence of new ways of conducting research (e.g., Spivak, 1993; Scheurich, 1995; St Pierre, 1997; St Pierre & Pillow, 2000), adopting the names of 'post-inquiry' and/or 'post-qualitative research'. Here, I will use the second descriptor because of its immediate link to qualitative research.

It would be inaccurate to describe post-qualitative research as a new methodology because, at its core, it is the difficult and laudable aspiration to free the researcher as much as possible from the constraints of methodology. For that reason, post-qualitative research is animated by a creative tension: on the one hand, challenging the limitations of both quantitative and qualitative research methodologies, and on the other, holding the new emerging ideas lightly enough so that they do not become new formulae and/or constraints.

This up-and-coming *non*-methodology has yet to reach the world of psychotherapy. My attempt here is to communicate some of the ontological and epistemological aspects of post-qualitative research in the hope that the latter may be included in psychotherapy trainings and that it may begin to inform some of our thinking as clinicians.

Paradigm wars (and treaties)

As a rule, psychotherapy research within most theoretical orientations tends to outline clear differences between quantitative and qualitative methodologies (often, but not always, privileging the latter). While the former has a long history, dating back to the early years of the 20th century and the logical positivism of the Vienna Circle, the latter is relatively new, with the first volume of the journal *Qualitative Inquiry* being published in the mid-1990s. There are crucial distinctions between the two modalities, the most obvious being *primary* and *secondary* distinctions:

- *Primary* distinction relates to the production of data and the nature of indicators: numbers in the case of quantitative research; words in the case of qualitative

DOI: 10.4324/9781003669906-6

research. A research is then labelled 'mixed-methods' research when it succeeds in presenting and discussing both quantitative (numbers) and qualitative (words) indicators.

- *Secondary* distinction relates to epistemological assumptions, i.e. with the style of propositions by which researchers formulate their understanding of what constitutes knowledge, usually in relation to existing theories. How do we know what we know? How do we articulate it? Do we, for instance, devise or rely on *causal* explanations, apportioning origins, finding certitude in ascribing purpose, unity and reason to the phenomena we study? Do we perceive them as external, solid objects from an imaginary vantage-point? Do we, in other words, apply a *positivist* explanation? Or do we instead approach phenomena through empathic attunement, our 'garment' becoming so thoroughly 'invisible' that we may ourselves forget we are wearing it? Do we, in other words, apply a *hermeneutical* explanation?

If we adhere to the above distinctions, the two modes of enquiry appear to be incompatible, with the quantitative and qualitative divider becoming all the more marked, positing objectivity against subjectivity, being against becoming, static against flowing and so forth. This has vital implications for psychotherapy. Consider, for instance, Carl Rogers' well-known definition of the 'person' as a 'fluid process [rather than] a fixed and static entity; [as a] a flowing river of change, not a block of solid material; [as] a continually changing constellation of potentialities, not a fixed quantity of traits' (Rogers, 1961, p. 122). This fluid perspective is seemingly incompatible with a positivistic, quantitative stance, and more in step with an empathically attuned, qualitative stance. Understood in this way, the marked difference between the two modalities goes a long way towards explaining the vigorous 'paradigm wars' (Gage, 1989, p. 135) of a few decades ago, whose effects are arguably still present today. Various attempts have been made in recent years within the person-centred approach (PCA) to bridge the two modalities, with several practitioners leaning, surprisingly, in favour of quantitative methods. However, what these stances may ignore is the *political* element implicit in quantitative methodologies. Positivistic, quantitative ontologies and epistemologies have historically provided the ideological backdrop for and have enjoyed full patronage from, institutional power (whose agendas are altogether at variance, to put it mildly, from the exploratory and emancipatory enterprise of therapy), justifying the label of 'quantitative imperialism' (Brady & Collier, 2004, p. 15) that some authors attributed to it.

The empathetic stance found in qualitative research has been forcibly quashed in recent years through the impositions of fixed rules and standards, something which may be understood as a reflection of the turn, at the beginning of the 1980s, from the managed market economy and rational micro-economic level actions of Keynesian liberalism (1945–80) to neoliberalism, a mode first implemented by General Augusto Pinochet in Chile before becoming common currency the world over, and characterized by unbridled individualism and the rhetoric of 'natural' free markets.

Waiting for Rogers at the wrong station

The ideological pull of logical positivism which took hold first in Europe and then in the United States when members of the Vienna Circle fled Germany is not to be underestimated; it has been called the epistemological unconscious (Steinmetz, 2005). To be uncritically sympathetic, as person-centred/experiential practitioners, to quantitative methods means to turn a blind eye to the political pressures on psychotherapy on behalf of an audit culture of 'accountability' to bend to positivist agendas. To promote basic empathy scales, authenticity scales and related attempts to measure, translate and subjugate the subtleties and vagaries of human life means overlooking that a *number* is a *signifier like any other* (Bazzano, 2020), rather than a privileged signifier. We would be operating under the influence of what Andrew Natsios (2010) calls 'Obsessive Measurement Disorder' – a 'pathology' that has invaded not only government policies but also the humanities, including the therapy world. We would be waiting for Carl Rogers at the wrong station.

In wanting to bridge essentially qualitative endeavours such as person-centred/experiential therapies to a quantitative *modus operandi*, we would nevertheless affirm, albeit by accident, something important. We would be saying that there may be *no fundamental distinction* between quantitative and qualitative methods. Could that be true? And in what way can one make that claim?

In a paper on psychotherapy research in relation to language and gesture, Julia Cayne (2020) wrote about 'approaches to qualitative phenomenological research… as stemming from the dominant discourse around a positivist paradigm' (Internet file). Cayne's is a surprising statement: qualitative methods may well be at heart positivistic, just as quantitative methods are, despite the differences in their respective languages. Why? Because they may be a way, she goes on to say, to 'maneuver us *around experience* rather than recognize how we are *subject to*, in this case, language and importantly language as bodily phenomena' (emphases added). Within qualitative methods, she goes on to add, primacy is still given to universal truths, rather than the contextual, temporal, cultural' dimensions (Cayne, 2020, emphases added).

A few years ago, I would have balked at the very idea of fathoming a positivist continuum between quantitative and qualitative methodologies. My default had always been to instinctively defend the qualitative ethos against the onslaught of what I consider as mind-numbing and dehumanizing metrics. However, after years of learning and subsequently teaching research methods, I began to feel disillusioned with conventional humanistic qualitative methods, and increasingly unhappy about my own need to justify them. Part of the problem, I now realize with hindsight, was that I had studied post-structuralism long *before* embarking on a person-centred psychotherapy training whose tenets relied on a set of philosophical assumptions harking back to modernism. It has been somewhat comforting to learn of others who had gone through a similar process (e.g. St Pierre, 2014).

My own experience as both a trainee and trainer, and that of many of my colleagues, suggests that the ethos reigning over therapy trainings (including person-centred ones) is the preservation and perpetuation of a set of existing canonical tenets rather than genuine questioning. In my view, to encourage the latter would shake the foundation of an edifice painstakingly built to appease the powers; it would also put future funding at risk. When so-called 'universal' and metaphysical truths (whether coated in numbers, words or images, relying on a formative tendency or the alleged friendliness of facts) take over the irredeemably *asymmetrical* and contingent aspects of, say, our case-study or particular topic of research. When the solidity, coherence and substantiality of the speaking subject (Foucault, 1970) are not scrutinized but leaves the self-unscathed. When codes of belief and shibboleths are invariably confirmed, then the claim that conventional qualitative research is still in the grip of positivism begins to gain traction.

Is there a way out of the impasse? One possible way is moving the goalposts by looking at post-qualitative research (Lather, 2013; St Pierre, 2014; Le Grange, 2016, 2018) and seeing what it may offer to the PCA and experiential therapies.

Post-qualitative research

> Transformation [is] very urgent, very difficult, and quite possible.
>
> (Foucault, 1988, p. 155)

Upholding an overall sympathetic and supportive stance towards the conventional qualitative style of conducting research is a valid stance, but is that enough? To make our home there may well mean turning qualitative inquiry into another stale formula routinely recycled from one generation of practitioners to the next. The implicit promise of *post-qualitative* research is that in its current 'birthing state' would allow for the openness and experimentation which psychotherapy training, practice and research all need in order to open new avenues of inquiry. In my view, this is preferable to the present situation within the PCA, with two main tendencies arguably wrestling for ascendancy: on the one hand, precious upholding of the conventionally humanistic tenets of the approach; on the other, insistent calls for a renewal which relies on a positivist ethos at variance with the soul of the approach. I believe the first one looks to the past, the second looks not so much to the future as to *an upgrade*.

The added potential benefit of post-qualitative research is that it can provide not only an engaging critique of quantitative and qualitative methods, but it can also point the way towards a *new epistemology*, inviting us to think differently about knowledge. In so doing, it may renew the original purpose of qualitative research, while maintaining a refreshingly tentative, exploratory ambience.

A note on ontology and epistemology in post-qualitative research

What would this new epistemology consist of? This is clearly work in progress, but a starting point would be a trenchant critique of epistemology (or theory of knowledge) itself. Critical theory is very helpful here. For Adorno and Horkheimer (1947/2002), at the heart of human desire for knowledge is fear:

> Humans believe themselves free of fear when there is no longer anything unknown. This has determined the path of demythologization.
>
> (p. 11)

Constructing a theory of knowledge is inevitably animated by our fear and anxiety of the unknown.

What is the alternative suggested by a post-qualitative stance? Not *abandoning* knowledge altogether but seeing it as a useful fiction, in the positive sense of the term, i.e. as a creative human endeavour that helps us to a degree to make sense of an unfathomable world. This is a useful antidote against dogmatism, for then the tenets of a psychotherapeutic approach are seen as descriptors, hypotheses to be tested, rather than as articles of faith.

The notion of ontology would also be revised, for then this branch of metaphysics dealing with the nature of being (the literal meaning of ontology) would be submitted to closer scrutiny in post-qualitative thought and research. The inspiration here is Carl Rogers himself, if we take seriously his claim that a person is 'a fluid process, not a fixed static entity, a flowing river of change, not a block of solid material; a continually changing constellation of potentialities, not a fixed quantity of traits' (Rogers, 1961, p. 122). In other words, there is no such thing as *being* (what ontology is preoccupied with) but only *becoming*. An 'ontology' of becoming is possible: a fluid, 'musical' ontology that observes and is loyal to processes and is animated by a process philosophy (Whitehead, 1978).

Post-structuralism and critical theory: identity and emancipation

There are different cultural and philosophical sources within the nascent post-qualitative 'movement'. The ones I personally draw from are post-structuralism and (aspects of) critical theory, in particular the work of Walter Benjamin (2002). Other sources on which post-qualitative practitioners tend to draw are posthumanism, speculative realism and the more fuzzy term 'postmodernism'. I find these links far less convincing and less useful to our purposes here. Unlike post-structuralism and critical theory (both emancipatory practices), postmodernism has effectively become the ideology of neoliberalism (Jameson, 2013, 2019). Here, I will briefly sketch salient points in post-structuralism and critical theory before going on to explore ways in which their insights may be applied to psychotherapy research.

Post-structuralism is the broad, expedient term given to a set of diverse philosophical practices emerging around the 1950s, mainly but not only in France, and reaching an extraordinary flowering in the 1960s and 1970s with the publication of pivotal works by authors such as Foucault, Derrida, Deleuze and Guattari, Kristeva, Blanchot, Lyotard, Cixous, Irigaray – to name a few. Inscribed within a wider political project of emancipation and engaged in active and often critical dialogue within the historical Left, these writings influenced politics, psychiatry, psychoanalysis, philosophy, art and science. Looming in the background were figures like Nietzsche, an important influence on post-structuralism, but also writers such as Merleau-Ponty, de Beauvoir and Sartre, with whom post-structuralists engaged critically and creatively. Simply put, post-structuralist texts provide us, among other things, with a formidable *critique of identity*.

Critical theory, from its heyday of the early Frankfurt School (particularly Adorno and Benjamin) to Judith Butler and Eve Sedgwick, provides us first of all with a useful correlate to the above, namely the tools needed to formulate an *ontology of actuality*. To see through the insubstantiality of the self is not enough. Foucault (1983) acknowledged that many theoretical blunders could have been avoided in post-structuralism by paying closer attention to the *ontology of actuality* that runs through the Frankfurt School (Dews, 1986). Interestingly, contemporary expressions of social change and direct action such as the Occupy Wall Street movement did not turn to humanistic thought for inspiration, but to critical theory (Jeffries, 2016). What does 'ontology of actuality' mean? Wedding our actions to history and the everyday alongside concrete others.

I have for some time now discussed the importance of Hegel's *Phenomenology* (1977) in relation to therapy trainings (e.g. Bazzano, 2012, 2016a, 2017), highlighting the realities of conflict and disparity which need to be acknowledged alongside more popular and romanticized notions of mutuality and symmetry in relational psychotherapy. This point was developed further in my recent book (Bazzano, 2019) where the notion of actuality is grounded in the primacy of the *deed* at the expense of a frequently glorified *doer*. One important implication of this is a critique of intentionality – a staple ingredient in humanistic and phenomenological trainings – in favour of *expression*. This may be rightly construed as a call to *expressionism in psychotherapy*. Subjectivation in this context becomes *heterology*, or logic of the other (which also implies *primacy* of the other). My 'identity' – its 'imprint' – is clarified through expression and action (the domain of history, ethics, of finite, embodied existence) with others. It cannot be mere assertion of subjectivity. Emancipation then becomes political subjectivation, i.e. the formation of an identity that is not a 'self' but a concrete, conflictual/loving relation of self/others.

Applications

Person-centred, experiential and other psychotherapy trainings would benefit from exposure to post-structuralist and critical theory's texts as required reading. What would this mean in terms of research? What key points can be outlined? I will sketch a few, drawing mainly on Le Grange (2018).

- ***De-centering of the 'I'***. In post-qualitative research, the human 'I' is 'ecological, embedded in the material flows of the earth/cosmos, constitutive of these flows' (Le Grange, 2016, p. 34). It is never isolated from the three ecologies – mental, social, environment (Guattari, 2000). A de-centring of the speaking subject is 'crucial in an organismic perspective such as the PCA' (Bazzano, 2012, p. 140). For Deleuze and Guattari (1987), the human is not separate but on an immanent plane with a world of materiality which, far from being inert matter, is gifted with *agency* (Bennett, 2010; Coole & Frost, 2010; Bazzano, 2012), i.e. with self-organizing (self-actualizing) capabilities.

- ***Re-envisioning epistemology***. Excessive importance is given to knowledge in both quantitative and qualitative methodologies. The latter may at times criticize knowledge, but it still continues to attach great importance to it. Despite nominally critiquing the Cartesian *cogito* (the thinking 'I'), it still holds on to the knowledge gained by 'my' research. Also, not enough attention is paid to the close proximity and even complicity of knowledge to institutional power and, among other things, to the links 'between knowledge and ethics [and] how knowledge produces reality' (St Pierre, 2013, p. 648).
- ***Non-representational research***. Both quantitative and qualitative methodologies rely on logocentrism, i.e. the view, central in Western science and philosophy, which assumes the existence of a fundamental unity between language and reality. They also tend to condense difference, fragmentation and subjectivity into a larger, all-encompassing whole that often relies on logic and reason, and the allegedly unifying structure of language. The post-qualitative researcher goes beyond this view, attempting a non-representational mode of research, which Ingold (2015, p. vii) explains as

  > a *correspondence*, in the sense of not coming up with some exact match or simulacrum for what we find in the things and happenings going on around us, but of *answering* them with interventions, questions and responses of our own. (original emphases)

- ***Pure experience***. Here, the invitation is to go beyond the crushing dullness of codes and categories. In both quantitative and qualitative data analysis, the researcher examines 'data' as an object out there, separated from them. This implies 'violence to thought' (Deleuze, 2000/1964, p. 97) and can be resisted in post-qualitative research. The inspiration here draws from radical empiricism. Erin Manning (2015) explains:

  > The challenge of radical empiricism is that it begins in the midst of relations not yet organized into terms such as 'subject' and 'object'. William James calls this field of relations 'pure experience', pure understood not in the sense of 'purity' but in the sense of immanent to actual relations. Pure experience is on the cusp of the virtual and the actual: in the experiential register of the not-quite yet. It is of experience in the sense that it affectively contributes to how experience settles into what James calls 'knower–known' relations. As with Deleuze's actual–virtual distinction, pure experience is the in-folding of potential that keeps actual experience open to its more-than. (p. 55)

An evocative way to articulate this 'anti-method' stance in relation to so-called data is found in Lather (2013). We are invited to 'make love to' rather than analyse our data:

> Making love to one's data becomes thinkable as a kind of ethics, something quite different from 'better or smarter', something more akin to the in-between places of pleasure and pain. Struggling with and against, becoming more and other, 'in a field of production of desire', analysis moves way beyond interpretation.
>
> (Lather, 2013, p. 639)

- *Axiology*. I believe this is central to psychotherapy (Bazzano, 2019), and as such it merits a brief explication here. Axiology (from *axioein*, to 'hold worthy') is the science of ascribing *values* to phenomena: in the context of therapy, this means determining the balance of *active* and *reactive* forces in the organism. A force is active when it is allowed to do what it can do. A force becomes reactive when, diverted by extraneous (usually normative) concerns, it turns against itself. An example of an active force is as any micro-disposition – emotion, feeling, instinct, affect etc. – which is trusted enough to be allowed to 'do its thing' and reveal the inherent wisdom and innocence within an overall tendency to act itself out – or *actualize*. Conversely, a reactive force is that very same micro-disposition mistrusted, judged and turned against its own natural momentum (in the name, for example, of a strong and unchallenged external locus of evaluation). The task of psychotherapy is then to work in the service of active forces, facilitating (organismic) actualization, and further advancing Rogers' central recognition of 'life [as] an *active* process, not a passive one', a recognition that 'the behaviors of an organism move in the direction of maintaining, enhancing and reproducing itself'. 'Enhancing' is the key word here; when working in the service of active forces, we affirm the life of the organism as an expansive force revelling in the sheer pleasure of knowing itself differently through its individualized expression. Arguably, this is wholly different from attempts to measure, regulate and ultimately control the life force of an organism in the service of the dominant ideologies and the market.

As for drawing from critical theory, the other influence behind the present article, I will limit myself to sketch a few key ideas drawn from Walter Benjamin (2002), the first of which draws, interestingly, from medieval theology. A brief premise will be in order here.

My own experience as a writer taught me that it is only *after* the deed, as it were – with the book written, the paper assembled, the article done and a stumbling but eager *corpus* growing in the psychical shed – that I found more direct resonance, or rather reverberation, with the work of Walter Benjamin and his own bungling attempts at research. The finding was accidental. I had turned to Benjamin for entirely different reasons – for reasons similar to those of Italian philosopher Giorgio Agamben who was looking for an 'antidote' that would allow him 'to survive Heidegger' (de la Durantaye, 2009, p. 53). On a spring day in 1940, Benjamin handed to librarian Georges Bataille at the *Biblioteque Nationale* in Paris a gigantic manuscript on Baudelaire. In it, he comments on topics as many and varied as allegory, alienation, philosophy, poetry in the age of advanced capitalism and some intriguing notions such as 'the now of knowability' and 'love at last sight', the fleeting nature of love in the modern metropolis. His friend Theodor Adorno, after reading the manuscript, criticized what he judged to be a wide-eyed presentation of mere facticity. Benjamin took that as a compliment, saying something to the effect of 'you are describing the proper philological attitude'.

- ***Forma Fluens.*** What is then 'Benjamin's method'? And why do I find it so congenial? In Benjamin (2002), inspiration comes from a notion already present in medieval theology, according to which *forma fluens*, the flowing shape of matter, is organized by the force of divine intellect. Adorno had been rightly concerned that the view expounded by his friend was too mystical and non-dialectical. In their correspondence of 12 years (1928–40), Benjamin (2002) explains that it is not divine intellect that does the organizing but 'our own historical experience'. And here is the crucial point: matter itself – what contemporary thought calls 'materiality', i.e. beyond inert 'matter' (Bennett, 2010; Coole & Frost, 2010; Bazzano, 2012) – assembles and 'actualizes' without the intervention of either a demiurge or its shadows and surrogates, whether 'Being' or a 'Truth' that one expects to unveil. This process of autonomous construction also belongs to what we call in our psych trade 'research'. Construction is not imposed in the aftermath of data analyses; it emerges from its own intimate/immanent movement, which is how Benjamin conducted his own bungling and inspired research. Interested in just about everything, looking at every corner for emancipatory possibilities, he personified the distant travels of philosophy outside its arbitrary borders and fences. Could this way of conducting research be what phenomenology is in its purest sense? Probably not, if we consider that phenomenology is inevitably mired in subjectivism, despite the best efforts by Merleau-Ponty to at least posit a '*body*-subject'.

Lather and Kitchens (2017) have brilliantly outlined other key points which draw on Benjamin and can be useful to post-qualitative research. I will summarize and adapt some of them below, in no particular order, adding some of my own:

- *Reading ('data') against ourselves.* This is akin to what in Zen we call 'beginner's mind' and what I have myself called the stance of the 'therapist as idiot' (Bazzano, 2016b). It implies resisting the compulsion to mastery and reduction to one point of view in favour of contradiction, movement and uncertainty (Lather & Kitchens, 2017).
- *Giving primacy to 'becoming'*: focusing on surprises, incongruities, novelties, repetitions. Paying great attention to cracks, contradictions without turning the 'material' into linear, logical narratives.
- *Becoming an unreliable researcher.* This implies outright refusal of official knowledge and of the alleged power of the reporter/chronicler, alongside a resistance to what the 'truth' of our findings might be. This point acknowledges

that the truth we tell ourselves and others at the most is expedient, utilitarian and subject to change.

- *Paying attention to how we tell a story.* Whether writing a case-study, investigating racism in therapy trainings, or writing about dream work, we could do well to notice how we put together a story, what we exclude and why, what we deem irrelevant, unacceptable, embarrassing etc.
- *Establishing a sacred-cow-free zone.* This relates to engaging deeply with our sources, including and especially texts of our particular approach/tribe/parish, noticing how they speak to us, making room for critique. The latter is another word for freedom, which is essential in research.
- *'Weighing up' our sources.* As with the earlier discussion on axiology, here the question is: 'Does the source I'm drawing on express an expansive, life-affirming, emancipatory ethos?'

Many things (virtually everything) can and should be deconstructed in post-qualitative research. For example: the *interview* (Scheurich, 1995), *authenticity, empathy* (Lather, 2000), and reflexivity (Pillow, 2003) can all be ousted and re-thought, thus making space for the new.

A guide to getting lost

Keeping psychotherapy research alive and able to respond to ever-changing contingencies means in many ways getting lost (Solnit, 2006), rather than getting knowledgeable, unless one understands, with Plato, knowledge as love, in which case knowledge *is* getting lost – losing oneself, relinquishing the Cartesian 'I' and drowning happily in the waters of our so-called data, making love to our data and be forever changed by them beyond repair. Emancipatory psychotherapies can no longer sheepishly rely on the tired and trite tenets of quantitative and conventional qualitative methods. The organism seeks greater actualization. What the latter looks and feels like is not a given or a pre-existing idea but is experienced/experimented with the crucible of practice, in the midst of unpredictable contingencies. Post-qualitative research sketches a possible way out of our current impasse.

Bibliography

Adorno, T. W. & Horkheimer, M. (1947/2002). *Dialectic of Enlightenment: Philosophical Fragments.* Stanford, CA: Stanford University Press.

Bazzano, M. (2012). Immanent vitality: reflections: on the actualizing tendency, *Person Centered and Experiential Psychotherapies*, 11 (2): 137–151.

Bazzano, M. (2016a). The conservative turn in person-centered therapy. *Person Centered and Experiential Psychotherapies*, 15 (4): 339–355.

Bazzano, M. (2016b). The therapist as idiot. *Hermeneutic Circular*, April: 10–11.

Bazzano, M. (2017). *Zen and Therapy: Heretical Perspectives.* Abingdon: Routledge.

Bazzano, M. (2019). *Nietzsche and Psychotherapy.* Abingdon: Routledge.

Bazzano, M. (2020). The skin is faster than the word. *Existential Analysis*, 31 (1): 53–64.

Benjamin, W. (2002). *Charles Baudelaire: un poeta lirico nell'etá del capitalismo avanzato.* Vicenza: Neri Pozza.

Bennett, J. (2010). *Vibrant Matter: A Political Ecology of Things*. Durham, NC: Duke University Press.

Brady, H. & Collier, D. (eds) (2004). *Rethinking Social Inquiry: Diverse Tools, Shared Standards*. Lanham, MD: Rowman & Littlefield.

Cayne, J. (2020). Language and gesture in Merleau-Ponty: some implications for method in therapeutic practice and research. *European Journal of Psychotherapy and Counselling*, 22 (1–2): 30–44.

Coole, D. & Frost, S. (eds) (2010). *New Materialisms: Ontology, Agency, and Politics.* Durham, NC: Duke University Press.

De la Durantaye, L. (2009). *Giorgio Agamben: A Critical Introduction.* Stanford, CA: Stanford University Press.

Deleuze, G. (2000). *Proust and Signs: The Complete Text*, trans. R. Howard. Minneapolis: University of Minnesota Press (orig publ 1964).

Deleuze, G. & Guattari, F. (1987). *A Thousand Plateaus: Capitalism and Schizophrenia.* Minneapolis: University of Minnesota Press.

Dews, P. (1986). Adorno, post-structuralism and the critique of identity. *New Left Review* I, 157: 28–44.

Foucault, M. (1970). *The Order of Things: An Archaeology of the Human Sciences.* New York: Vintage Books.

Foucault, M. (1983). Structuralism and post-structuralism: an interview with Michel Foucault. *Telos*, 55: 200.

Foucault, M. (1988). Technologies of the self. In L. H. Martin, H. Gutman, & P. H. Hutton (eds.), *Technologies of the Self: A Seminar with Michel Foucault* (pp. 16–49). Amherst: University of Massachusetts Press.

Gage, N. (1989). The paradigm wars and their aftermath: a 'historical' sketch of research on teaching since 1989. *Teachers College Record*, 91 (2): 135–150.

Guattari, F. (2000). *The Three Ecologies*. London: Athlone.

Hegel, G. W. F. (1977). *Phenomenology of Spirit.* Oxford: Oxford University Press (orig publ 1807; trans. A.V. Miller).

Ingold, T. (2015). Foreword. In P. Vannini (ed.), *Non-representational Methodologies: Re-visioning Research* (pp. vii–xx). London: Routledge.

Jameson, F. (2013). *The Antinomies of Realism*. London & New York: Verso.

Jameson, F. (2019). *Allegory and Ideology*. London & New York: Verso.

Jeffries, S. (2016). *Grand Hotel Abyss: The Lives of the Frankfurt School.* London: Verso.

Lather, P. (2000). Against empathy, voice and authenticity. *Women, Gender and Research* (Cophenhagen). (Special issue on Transgressive Methodology), 4: 16–25.

Lather, P. (2013). Methodology-21: what do we do in the afterward? *International Journal of Qualitative Studies in Education*, 26 (6): 634–645.

Lather, P. & Kitchens, J. (2017). Applied Benjamin: educational thought, research and pedagogy. *Journal of Curriculum Theorizing,* (32) 1; available at https://tinyurl.com/y6tkuspq (accessed 9 January 2021).

Lather, P. & St Pierre, E. A. (2013). Post-qualitative research. *International Journal of Qualitative Studies in Education*, 26 (6): 629–633.

Le Grange, L. (2016). Sustainability education and (curriculum) improvisation. *Southern African Journal of Environmental Education*, 32: 26–36.

Le Grange, L. (2018). What is (post)qualitative research? *South African Journal of Higher Education*, 32 (5): 1–14.
Manning, E. (2015). Against method. In P. Vannini (ed.), *Non-representational Methodologies: Re-visioning Research* (pp. 52–71). London: Routledge.
Natsios, A. (2010). The clash of the counter-bureaucracy and development. *Center for Global Development*, 1 July; available at https://www.cgdev.org/content/publications/detail/1424271 (accessed 5 January 2020).
Pillow, W. S. (2003). Confession, catharsis, or cure? Rethinking the uses of reflexivity as methodological power in qualitative research. *International Journal of Qualitative Studies in Education,* 16 (2): 175–196.
Rogers, C. R. (1961). *On Becoming a Person.* London: Constable.
Scheurich, J. J. (1995). A postmodernist critique of research interviewing. *International Journal of Qualitative Studies in Education*, 8 (3): 239–252.
Solnit, R. (2006). *A Field Guide to Getting Lost.* London: Canongate.
Spivak, G. C. (1993). *Outside in the Teaching Machine.* New York: Routledge.
St Pierre, E. A. (1997). Methodology in the fold and the irruption of transgressive data. *International Journal of Qualitative Studies in Education*, 10 (2): 175–189.
St Pierre, E. A. (2013). The posts continue: becoming. *International Journal of Qualitative Studies in Education*, 26 (6): 646–657.
St Pierre, E. (2014). A brief and personal history of post-qualitative research: towards 'post inquiry'. *Journal of Curriculum Theorizing*, 30 (2): 2–19; available at https://tinyurl.com/y6cnculs (accessed 9 January 2021).
St Pierre, E. A. & Pillow, W. S. (eds) (2000). *Working the Ruins: Feminist Poststructural Theory and Methods in Educations.* New York: Routledge.
Steinmetz, G. (2005). The epistemological unconscious of U.S. sociology and the transition to post-Fordism: the case of historical sociology. In J. Adams, E. S. Clemens, & A. Shola Orloff (eds.), *Remaking Modernity: Politics, History, Sociology* (pp. 109–157). Durham, NC: Duke University Press.
Whitehead, A. N. (1978). *Process and Reality*. New York: The Free Press.

Chapter 6

Therapy beyond concepts

Direct experience and active forces in therapy

Dániel Ványi

Introduction

According to Bazzano (2023), there exists "a wider domain of experiencing, a *threshold* from which transformation may occur" (p. 80). He describes this mode of experiencing as not being fixated on the self or subject as the centre of experience, but instead taking on board a more diffuse perspective of phenomenal experiencing (see also Bazzano, 2017). Dews (1986) claims that subjectivity presupposes a conceptual representation of the experiencing self. In Gyamtso and Hookham's (1988) presentation of the Buddhist understanding of the mind, all our conceptualizations are founded on the fundamental illusion of separating the experiencing mind (subject) from the experienced objects. Whether we think that the subject (self) or concepts come first, the subject as the centre of experience is closely intertwined with conceptual abstractions of immediate experiencing (Dews, 1986; Gyamtso & Hookham, 1988; Trungpa & Guenther, 2003; Trungpa, 2002a, 2002b).

As opposed to the conceptual mode of experiencing, direct or nonconceptual experiencing is a form of experience that is not mediated by concepts – therefore, it is also not fixated on the (concept of) a self separate from experiencing (Gyamtso & Hookham, 1988; McLeod, 2001). In the following sections, I will examine the nature of this form of experiencing and outline some hypotheses about its possible role in therapy work.

Various traditions of thought differentiate between a direct or nonconceptual dimension of experience and conceptual-theoretical constructions (abstractions of direct experience). The distinction exists, for example, in phenomenology, post-structuralism, analytic philosophy, cognitive science and also in the traditional Buddhist understanding of the mind and experience. Of course, the distinction is not absolute, since, on one level, concepts are also part of the flux of immediate experiencing, but on another level, a qualitative difference exists between concept-mediated and direct or nonconceptual experiencing (Bazzano, 2009, 2019; Gyamtso & Hookham, 1988). There is a difference between experiencing concepts or thoughts as parts of the immediate flow of experience and experiencing *through* concepts.

DOI: 10.4324/9781003669906-7

Phenomenology is a philosophical approach particularly interested in direct experience. Phenomenological psychologist William James (1904, see also Goodman, 2004) differentiated between the flow or "quasi-chaos" of experience – he also called it pure experience – and concepts that dissect this "quasi-chaos" into separate, seemingly solid entities. Merleau-Ponty (1945/2013) talked about direct experience as the experience of things in themselves, as experience that precedes knowledge, experience that all knowledge is an abstraction of. According to Sinha (1963), "The slogan of phenomenological reduction is to go back 'to the things themselves' (…) as the immediate 'phenomena' (…) Phenomenological analysis (…) is not, as such, concerned with linguistic expressions, but with the phenomena within the region of immanent experience meant by such expressions" (pp. 571–572). These are some examples of describing direct or nonconceptual experience in the phenomenological tradition.

Deleuze and Guattari (1994) talked about *the plane of immanence*, a prephilosophical, preconceptual or nonconceptual plane that "constitutes the absolute ground of philosophy… the foundation on which it creates its concepts" (p. 41). Since, for them, the beginning of philosophy is the creation of concepts, the plane of immanence is the prephilosophical ground of philosophy. As they explain, "It is presupposed not in the way that one concept may refer to others but in the way that concepts themselves refer to a nonconceptual understanding" (Deleuze & Guattari, 1994, p. 40).

The notion of nonconceptual or direct experiencing – under various names – is central in *Tibetan Buddhism* and the closely related *Dzogchen* teachings. Tibetan Buddhist teacher Chogyam Trungpa talked about "shunyata" or "emptiness" as "an experiential reality which can never be accurately described because words simply are not the experience. Words or concepts only point to partial aspects of experience. In fact, it is dubious that one can even speak of "experiencing" reality, since this would imply a separation between the experiencer and the experience. Thus, the Madhyamika school simply speaks of the tathata, "as it is" (p. 191). In Trungpa and Guenther's common work (2003), this is called "peak experience" and is described as "an experience in which all conceptions and judgments, even the idea of oneself, completely pass away" (p. 345). Dzogchen teacher James Low talks about "a direct experience that words cannot really convey – it is not constructed out of concepts" (Dorje & Low, 2004, p. 103). Gyamtso and Hookham (1988) describe the nonconceptual Wisdom Mind (as understood in the Shentong school of Tibetan Buddhism) as

> empty of the conceptual process of distinguishing outer perceived objects as different in substance to the inner perceiving minds… It is completely free from any conceptualizing process and knows in a way that is completely foreign to the conceptual mind. It is completely unimaginable in fact.
>
> (p. 84)

Direct experience in therapy?

The idea that direct or nonconceptual experience might be important for therapy work occurred to me when reading Bazzano's definition of non-directivity in his book titled *Zen and Therapy* (2017). There, he differentiates two aspects of non-directivity – an essential attitude for the free exploration of experience. The first aspect is an "ethical respect for the client's autonomy and an expression of dynamic faith in the human being's inner resources", and the second aspect is "the aspiration to suspend explanations about reality, allowing space to notice emergent phenomena: a registering of experience devoid of a centre, a loyalty to non-centred experience" (p. 130). He continues explaining that "The imposition of a logically organized view of reality is prescriptive rather than descriptive and betrays a misunderstanding of sunyata" (p. 130). A closely related concept in person-centred therapy is the notion of presence. In his later work, Carl Rogers (1980) described *presence* as an important aspect of therapy work, and he defined it as being in touch with the unknown, intuitive and non-rational aspects of oneself. This idea was further explored by Geller and Greenberg (2002), who, based on interviews with therapists, clarified attributes of presence. One of the attributes they described was "approaching the client with an attitude of openness, interest, acceptance, and non-judgment rather than through the lens of preconceived knowledge or beliefs" (p. 77). They pointed out that many therapists associated this quality with meditation practice and Buddhism: "A therapist described the experience of therapeutic presence itself as akin to a meditative state or being aware or mindful" (p. 77). Another attribute of presence suggested by Geller and Greenberg was a non-attached attitude, in the sense of "letting go of control of what will be experienced... or even of the outcome of the therapy" (2002, p. 80). This understanding of presence seems to be very close to the notion of direct or nonconceptual experiencing. As Bazzano (2017) points out,

> Presence is understood in humanistic psychology as a way of being rather than the acquisition of a set of techniques, yet there are methods we can use in order to invite more presence in the therapy room and be helpful to our clients. In this sense, presence can be seen as a discipline inspired by the dimension of play. *It prepares the therapist to meet the unknown, the pre-cognitive and the pre-reflexive – the genuinely new.*
>
> (p. 63, italics added)

He further describes the present moment as being "fundamentally *unknowable* and strange" (Bazzano, 2019, p. 157).

While Rogers, Geller and Greenberg highlight presence/nonconceptual experience from the therapist's point of view, Purton (2004) explains that it is also important in the therapy process for the client to access this nonverbal, nonconceptual, "implicit" dimension. Bazzano (2017) emphasizes that presence is not the exclusive province of the therapist and it is mutually constituted.

Direct experience of therapist and client

The Buddhist notion of *transmission* is key to the teacher-student relationship in this tradition. According to Ken McLeod's (2001), explanation of the meaning of transmission lies in the fact that a person's presence opens up the possibility of presence in those around him or her. In Buddhism, they often refer to presence as synonymous with direct or nonconceptual experiencing: for Mcleod (2001), the practice of presence means "to be present with experience as it arises without trying to analyze it, understand it conceptually, or change it in any way" (p. 34). So, according to the Buddhist tradition, if someone is present in this sense of experiencing without conceptual understanding, this might facilitate this way of experiencing for other peope around them. I think this might be an important aspect of transformative therapeutic work.

A similar view was expressed by Chogyam Trungpa (2005), when he gave talks about the role of psychologists in therapy. According to him, it is important for the therapist to be connected to their own "basic sanity" – as he sometimes called the immediate, nonconceptual nature of experience – in order to be able to help their clients access the same fundamental sanity in their own minds. He explained that this way of experiencing is essential for genuine and compassionate communication. He also emphasized the importance of meditation practice for therapists in order to be able to access this nonconceptual perspective. He went as far as suggesting that Buddhism could revolutionize Western psychology by offering the perspective of the primacy of immediate experience and the method of meditation to access it, since these had been missing from this discipline.

Active and reactive forces, affect and transformation

So far, I have set up the hypothesis that the direct or nonconceptual mode of experiencing is relevant for therapy work, and that the therapist's ability to access this perspective might open up the possibility for the client as well to connect with it. Now I would like to link these ideas to the notions of active forces, affect and transformation. In short, I believe that direct experiencing may facilitate a free manifestation of affect and active forces in the psyche, and in turn, this opens up the possibility of a deeper psychic and social-cultural transformation.

The notions of affect, active and reactive forces and transformation are based on what is called the philosophical *counter-tradition*. From this perspective, the aim of philosophy, theory and research is not to *know* reality, in the sense of representing it or gaining a correct or true understanding of it, but instead, to actively participate in reality in the service of active, emancipatory forces (Bazzano, 2021a, 2021b; Madison, 1991; Ingold, 2015). Since reality is a flux, a constant flow of change or becoming, it is not even possible to create a correct representation of it: it changes every moment (Bazzano, 2017, 2019). In other words, there is no fixed or stable truth. Grosz (2017) points out beautifully how this perspective entails that ontology – an account of what is real – cannot be separated from ethical and political matters:

> insofar as we create ontologies that reflect not only, or primarily, beings but also becomings… an ontoethics cannot but address the question of how to act in the present and, primarily, how to bring about a future different from the present. This question is simultaneously ontological, ethical, and political.
>
> (p. 1)

Therefore, a bridge is formed from philosophy to practice, including therapeutic practice.

According to Bazzano (2019), a psychotherapeutic practice inspired by counter-traditional – and more specifically Nietzschean and Deleuzean philosophy – would focus on the dynamics of active versus reactive forces and favour/support the power of active forces in human psyche and culture: "A force is active when it is allowed to do what it can do. A force becomes reactive when, diverted by what Rogers calls an external locus of evaluation, it turns against itself" (Bazzano, 2021b, p. 44). Reactive forces maintain the status quo, protect existing identities and adapt to circumstances (Bazzano, 2019, 2023). In contrast, active forces are subversive: they break down structures, mechanisms of control, conceptual schemas and theories about the self and the world. They put into question the power of the self to control experience. They are pre-subjective, impersonal natural forces (Bazzano, 2023), which makes them resonate with the "neutral intensity of affect" (Bazzano, 2019, p. 61).

Affect theory is a recent manifestation of the philosophical counter-tradition. According to Bazzano (2023), "affect is the pre-verbal, impersonal flow of life's intensity and immediacy traversing living organisms" (p. 231). It is a domain beyond representation, discourse or reason (Bazzano, 2013a, 2016; Cronan, 2012) – therefore nonconceptual in nature. Affect is not the same as emotion. Emotion implies that the intensity of affect has been captured by conceptualization – "socio-linguistic fixation" – and made personal (Massumi, 1995). Affect is closely related to the body. In fact, it has been defined as the power of bodies to affect and be affected (Seigworth & Gregg, 2010). It is a "processual engagement of becoming" with no clear differentiation of subject and object (Seigworth & Gregg, 2010, p. 12). We can never know in advance what affect is capable of becoming (Hardt, 2007), so it connects us to the unexpected, the unknown, the ineffable – the nonconceptual. It is linked to the feeling of being alive (Clough, 2007).

Bazzano (2019) argues that in modern culture, reactive forces have become dominant over active forces. This manifests in many phenomena, from the hegemony of neopositivism in science and the profit-above-all attitude of neoliberal thinking, to the over-emphasizing of conscious rationality, control, security and the *ego-self* in psychology. Rogers also talked about the overdominance of rationality and control in different spheres of our society, including politics and mainstream psychotherapy. His notion of the actualizing tendency also resonates with the concept of active forces, although it is more easily (mis)read as unitary and having a predetermined goal, whereas active forces are clearly plural and lack a preconceived destination.

Active forces might instigate personal and cultural-societal transformations (Bazzano, 2019, 2023). Transformation is a process of radical change, the result of which cannot be known in advance and cannot be grasped by pre-existing concepts (Butler, 2004; Bazzano, 2013b). It involves the recognition that "we don't know who we are or what motivates us" (Bazzano, 2023, p. 122), that "the self is other to itself and ever-changing" (Bazzano, 2023, p. 131). Opening up to the power of active forces and the transformation they may bring about requires us to let go of our fixation to our idea of who we think we are: "The unitary subject gets in the way of transformation. What produces transformation is "a play of forces…". The *new* emerges as "a result of an activity that precedes the knowing subject…" (Bazzano, 2023, citing Butler, 2004, pp. 118–119). According to Butler (2004), for transformation to happen, we need to "disrupt what has become settled knowledge and knowable reality" (p. 27). This clearly resonates with the idea that the nonconceptual way of experiencing can facilitate transformation.

Nonconceptual experience and spontaneous energy

Tibetan Buddhist and Dzogchen teachers have talked about a freely flowing, spontaneous energy of the mind that is not bound by concepts as opposed to the conceptual channelling or controlling of energy performed by the ego (Trungpa, 2001, 2011; Dowman & Urgyen, 2008). In this approach, letting go of conceptual understanding makes it possible for us to open up to the basic, nonconceptual energy of wakefulness. In other words, the energy or intensity of emotions (feelings) can be experienced purely without conceptual/narrative interpretation (Chödrön, 2012). This nonconceptual yet wakeful energy is described as transcending the subject-object division (Urgyen, 2021). It resonates with the notion of affect as the preverbal, impersonal flow of life's intensity as well as the notion of active forces as pre-subjective, impersonal natural forces.

Although the spontaneous energy of wakefulness in Tibetan Buddhism is a wakeful (aware) energy and affect and active forces are characterized as unconscious in nature (Seigworth & Gregg, 2010; Deleuze, 1986), this is not necessarily a contradiction. Rational-conceptual (reactive) consciousness can be differentiated from a nonconceptual but aware quality of the mind (Dalai Lama, 2000, 2016; Dowman, 2020). As the Dalai Lama (2016) explains,

> For instance, you hear a noise, between the time of hearing it and conceptualizing its source, you can sense a state of mind that is devoid of thought but not asleep, in which the object is a reflection of the mind's luminosity and knowing. At such a point, the basic nature of the mind can be grasped.
>
> (p. 21)

As discussed above, this state of mind is also devoid of the differentiation between subject and object of experience (Gyamtso & Hookham, 1988; McLeod, 2001). This resonates with Deleuze's (2001) notion of an immanent *consciousness* that goes beyond the subject and the object, "a pure stream of a-subjective consciousness, a pre-reflexive impersonal consciousness, a qualitative duration of consciousness without a self" (p. 16).

Therefore, affect and active forces can be understood as unconscious only in the first sense, i.e. from the point of view of rational-conceptual consciousness. But they are not necessarily unconscious or unaware from the point of view of nonconceptual awareness. Nonconceptual experience itself might be understood as unconscious from the point of view of rational consciousness, since the latter cannot grasp it at all.

According to Bazzano (2017), "affect is a realm of experience not readily accessible through facts and reason, but one that may be approached by means of a more diffuse awareness" (p. 151). This also suggests that experiencing affect does not exclude some form of *awareness*. Cronan (2012) talks about "precognitive modes of awareness that were felt to be more basic, even more real than the ideated forms of linguistic apprehension" and cites Gibbs, who says that "affects constitute a 'level of experience [that] cannot be translated into words…'" (p. 51).

Furthermore, D. T. Suzuki (1960, 2015) talks about the notion of "unconscious consciousness" in Zen. He explains:

> But as intellectual development takes place, as we grow up, the sense-domain is invaded by intellect and the naivety of sense-experience is lost… The mature man is now asked by Zen… to free himself of the intellectual conscious interference if he sincerely wishes to realize a life of freedom and spontaneity where such disturbing feelings as fear, anxiety, or insecurity have no room to assail him. When this liberation takes place, we have the "trained" unconscious operating in the field of consciousness. And we know what Bankei's "Unborn" or the Chinese Zen master's "everyday mind" is.
>
> (Suzuki, 1960, pp. 19–20)

Similarly, Bazzano (2017) explains that the task in both Zen practice and therapy is to bring the conscious and the unconscious closer to each other, by "awakening to the mysterious, ambivalent nature of our conscious experience through a process of defamiliarization" (p. 152). Importantly, this quest involves "an intensification of awareness" (Cooper, 2010, cited by Bazzano, 2017, p. 152).

Conclusion

The nonconceptual, spontaneous and awake energy of the mind (as explained in Tibetan Buddhism) can be translated into affect and active forces in counter-traditional psychotherapy's terms. Although affect/active forces can never be fully controlled by conceptual consciousness, the latter still attempts to control or even repress them in order to maintain its preconceptions. Deconstructing conceptual reference points – and accessing the nonconceptual mode of experiencing – can undo this controlling effort. Therefore, nonconceptual experiencing helps us to open up to the power of affect and active forces in the psyche. In turn, this opening facilitates transformation, which is the proclaimed goal of Bazzano's (2019, 2023) counter-traditional psychotherapeutic endeavour. Thus, from this perspective, non-conceptual or direct experiencing is an important aspect of therapy work.

Bibliography

Bazzano, M. (2009). Brave new worlding: A response to Ernesto Spinelli's practicing existential psychotherapy. *Existential Analysis*, 20, 9–19.

Bazzano, M. (2013a). Back to the future: From behaviourism and cognitive psychology to motivation and emotion. *Self & Society*, 40(2), 32–35.

Bazzano, M. (2013b). On becoming no one: Phenomenological and empiricist contributions to the person-centered approach. *Person-Centered and Experiential Psychotherapies*, 13, 250–258.

Bazzano, M. (2016). Why process is (almost) everything. *Existential Analysis*, 27(1), 352–356.

Bazzano, M. (2017). *Zen and therapy: Heretical perspectives*. Abingdon: Routledge.

Bazzano, M. (2019). *Nietzsche and psychotherapy*. Abingdon: Routledge.

Bazzano, E. (2021a). *Identity and emancipation: Towards a counter-traditional, philosophically-informed psychotherapy*. Doctoral dissertation, University of Roehampton.

Bazzano, M. (2021b). Making love to your data. *Therapy Today*, 32(2), 42–45.

Bazzano, M. (2023). *Subversion and desire: Pathways to transindividuation*. Abingdon: Routledge.

Bazzano, M., & Webb, J. (2016). Introduction. In M. Bazzano & J. Webb (Eds.), *Therapy and the counter-tradition: The Edge of philosophy* (pp. 16–20). Abingdon: Routledge.

Butler, J. (2004). *Undoing gender*. New York: Routledge.

Chödrön, P. (2012). *Living beautifully with uncertainty and change*. Boulder, CO: Shambhala Publications.

Clough, P. T. (2007). Introduction. In P. T. Clough & J. Halley (Eds.), *The affective turn: Theorizing the social* (pp. 1–33). Durham, NC: Duke University Press.

Cooper, P. (2010). *The Zen impulse and the psychoanalytic encounter*. Abingdon: Routledge.

Cronan, T. (2012). Radically private and pretty uncoded. *Radical Philosophy*, 172, 51–53.

Dalai Lama (2000). *Dzogchen: Heart essence of the great perfection*. Ithaca, NY: Snow Lion.

Dalai Lama (2016). *The heart of meditation: Discovering innermost awareness*. Boulder, CO: Shambala.

Deleuze, G. (1986). *Nietzsche and philosophy*. London: Continuum.

Deleuze, G. (2001). *Pure immanence: Essays on a life*. New York: Zone Books.

Deleuze, G., & Guattari, F. (1994). *What is philosophy?* New York: Columbia University Press.

Dews, P. (1986). Adorno, post-structuralism and the critique of identity. *New Left Review*, 157(1), 28–44.

Dorje, N., & Low, J. (2004). *Being right here*. Ithaca, NY: Snow Lion.

Dowman, K. (2020). *Dzogchen Nonmeditation*. Kathmandu: Dzogchen Now! Books.

Dowman, K., & Urgyen (2008). *Gyémántszerelem [Diamond Love]*. Budapest: Oddijána.

Geller, S. M., & Greenberg, L. S. (2002). Therapeutic presence: Therapists' experience of presence in the psychotherapy encounter. *Person-Centered & Experiential Psychotherapies*, 1(1–2), 71–86.

Goodman, R. B. (2004). James on the nonconceptual. *Midwest Studies in Philosophy*, 28, 137–148.

Grosz, E. (2017). *The incorporeal: Ontology, ethics, and the limits of materialism.* New York: Columbia University Press.

Gyamtso, K. T., & Hookham, S. K. (1988). *Progressive stages of meditation on emptiness.* Oxford: Longchen Foundation.

Hardt, M. (2007). Foreword: What affects are good for. In P. T. Clough & J. Halley (Eds.), *The affective turn: Theorizing the social* (pp. ix–xiii). Durham, NC: Duke University Press.

Ingold, T. (2015). Foreword. In P. Vannini (Ed.), *Non-representational methodologies* (pp. VII–X). New York: Routledge.

James, W. (1904). A world of pure experience. *The Journal of Philosophy, Psychology and Scientific Methods,* 1(20), 533–543.

Madison, G. B. (1991). Beyond seriousness and frivolity: A Gadamerian response to deconstruction. In H. J. Silverman (Ed.), *Gadamer and hermeneutics* (pp. 119–135). New York: Routledge.

Massumi, B. (1995). The autonomy of affect. *Cultural Critique,* 31(31), 83–109.

McLeod, K. (2001). *Wake up to your life: Discovering the Buddhist path of attention.* San Francisco, CA: HarperSanFranciso.

Merleau-Ponty, M. (1945/2013). *Phenomenology of perception.* Abingdon: Routledge.

Rogers, C. R. (1980). *A way of being.* Boston, MA: Houghton Mifflin.

Seigworth, G. J., & Gregg, M. (2010). An inventory of shimmers. In M. Gregg & G. J. Seigworth (Eds.), *The affect theory reader* (pp. 1–25). Durham, NC: Duke University Press.

Sinha, D. (1963). Phenomenology and positivism. *Philosophy and Phenomenological Research,* 23(4), 562–577.

Suzuki, D. T. (2015). *Selected works of DT Suzuki, Volume I: Zen.* Oakland: University of California Press.

Suzuki, D. T., Fromm, E., & De Martino, R. (1960). *Zen Buddhism and psychoanalysis.* New York: Harper & Brothers.

Trungpa, C. (2001). *Crazy wisdom.* Boulder, CO: Shambhala Publications.

Trungpa, C. (2002a). *Cutting through spiritual materialism.* Boulder, CO: Shambhala Publications.

Trungpa, C. (2002b). *The myth of freedom and the way of meditation.* Boulder, CO: Shambhala Publications.

Trungpa, C. (2005). *The sanity we are born with: A Buddhist approach to psychology.* Boulder, CO: Shambhala Publications.

Trungpa, C. (2011). *Work, sex, money: Real life on the path of mindfulness.* Boulder, CO: Shambhala Publications.

Trungpa, C., & Guenther, H. V. (2003). The Dawn of Tantra. In C. R. Gimian (Ed.), *The collected works of Chogyam Trungpa, Volume 4* (pp. 329–419). Boulder, CO: Shambala Publications.

Urgyen (2021). *Égtáncosok és Őrült Jógik [Skydancers and Crazy Yogis].* Budapest: Samadhi.

Chapter 7

The affect of living in a dream world from a Nietzschean perspective

Glenn Nicholls

Introduction

When I was a young boy, my mother often said to me, 'Glenn, you are living in a dream world'. Of course she was right, although her comment was not intended as an insight into the reality of existence, it was an expression of concern. The unintended wisdom of her words was lost on me. I only came to appreciate the irony later when, according to her, I was too old to still be living in a dream world. Fortunately for me, I had also realised there is no age limit to living in the magical, fairy-tale world of dreams.

This chapter draws upon a recent road rage incident myself and another man witnessed and how it affected us both. I will describe how storytelling, having feelings and emotions and gaining self-knowledge can be little more than a defence against affect. I then describe how having 'open curiosity' (rather than 'closed curiosity') is necessary to better appreciate the primacy of affect. I explore how affect has a 'de-centring' and 'dispersive' quality and how this is integral to becoming 'lucid'. I also explore how affect is an expression of (pre)personal morals.

As a psychotherapist, I find working with affect easier than writing about it since affect does not have to make sense. Not making sense tends to work better in the consulting room than it does in a book about psychotherapy. In general, psychotherapy books are thought to be better when they make sense, although this is not always the case. Working with affect in psychotherapy is easier partly because its pre-personal, unintentional and nonsense-making qualities tend to work better in conversation than they do when read from a book.

Rather than writing *about* affect, I intend to write *with* it. Affect is necessarily affecting, though not by intention – affect has no intention. I *write for affect* in both senses, as an affirmation of life, and in order to have affect. Wanting to have affect is not the same as trying to effect someone or something. Since affect has no intention, writing for affect may appear as though I have put myself in a double-bind. This is not wholly the case since it is not possible to *cause* affect, since affect is not governed by the laws of cause and effect. A belief in cause and effect does not make affect subject to them, besides, I see cause and effect as, at best, a valuable illusion.

DOI: 10.4324/9781003669906-8

The law of cause and effect is the belief that effect is temporally preceded by cause and that one is distinct from the other. In other words, believing in cause and effect depends on a belief in time (which I also do not believe in). Affect does not require a belief in time since affect is non-temporal. Interestingly, time is a perfect example of the illusion of cause and effect insofar as the ending of a second appears to cause the next one to occur, and so on. Nonetheless, there is only affect *and* affect, and even then, it is not entirely possible to separate one from another, that said affect can sometimes be distinguished by its tonality and intensity.

Deleuze and Guattari's description of affect is helpful and problematic, they describe it as 'a pre-personal intensity corresponding to the passage from one experiential state of the body to another' (Deleuze & Guattari, 1987, p. xvi). This is helpful insofar as it grounds affect in the body, since, in a certain sense *affect constitutes the body*. It is somewhat problematic as it suggests that one state is distinct and separate from another, which is a similar sort of contrivance as the concept of time. While affect may be particular to an individual, it is not personal, nor is it trans-personal since it is experienced before it can become personal, making it pre-personal. In other words, it is there before the person exists, or, as we shall see later, affect brings them into existence.

Affect is not so much the medium through which we are able to experience our body, in a certain sense affect *is* the body: it is the experience of 'being' a body. Bodies can be described as *having* affect in the way the sun has rays, in other words, bodies cannot exist without affect. Another thing I like about Deleuze and Guattari's description is that it comes close to describing dream process. I will come onto the significance of this later.

One way of imagining affect is to picture two stringed instruments in a room, if one string vibrates, they all do. It is pointless asking from which string or instrument the vibration originated, if indeed it even came from within the room. Now picture the room with no walls, ceiling or floor. When I sit with people in psychotherapy the walls of my consulting room no longer exist, affect can come from anywhere manifesting in the room through the prism of conversation – or its absence.

While writing this chapter, I have noticed how, rather than writing a beginning, a middle and an end, I seem only able to write beginnings. This makes sense insofar as affect registers as *an opening*, and since affect has no end, there is no middle. Affect is like sound in that it changes in tonality and intensity, and even as it breaks, its silence has affect. As we go further into the chapter, a picture will emerge of the difference between the experience of affect and of telling a story about it. A story tends to have a beginning, a middle and an end, they also have a dramatic arc, affect has none of these. Affect can be experienced as an endless introduction as it opens us up and can keep us open.

Hugging a strange man

I recently witnessed a road rage incident with an unanticipated outcome. As I walked down a street, I saw two Arab men get out of separate cars to continue an aggressive confrontation with each other. Part of me wanted to shout at them to stop, but I knew that this would simply be joining in with them in their confrontation and their story. Instead, I allowed myself to experience the affect of the encounter before walking on. As I started to walk off, a man caught up to me. The man introduced himself as Sudanese and told me that he had also just witnessed the incident. He explained how the two men were from different Sudanese tribes, and that the altercation had more to do with tribal rivalry than anything else. The man said that he had followed me because he had noticed that as I watched them I had tears in my eyes. He wanted to hug me, he too had clearly been affected, I could see tears in his eyes.

I wondered what the man thought of our tears. On a superficial level, he saw a stranger from another culture, and although we were nobody to each other, we had tears in common. It struck me that it may be possible to have understanding without knowing what it is. Rather than thinking I knew what had affected either of us, or why he had followed me, by staying open to affect I had resisted the temptation of knowledge, and in so doing, we had inadvertently facilitated a different kind of encounter. The affect of our encounter and of witnessing the altercation was pre-personal, pre-feeling, pre-emotion, pre-knowledge and pre-story.

Feelings shape personal stories, whereas emotions shape social stories. The familiar stories we tell ourselves are also informed by another type of story, self-knowledge. What we know about ourselves and the world *is* a story. Stories can be wonderful – but are not fit for habitation, as soon as you are living in a story, wonder is lost. Thoughts, feelings and emotions overtake us as we get drawn into what happens next, and how the story will end.

As I walked away and before the man caught up with me, a sense of weariness came over me. I noticed how I began to interpret my experience as feelings and emotions, and as I did so I recognised how this experience was now reforming itself into an old familiar story, unwelcome and safe. The tears were neither feelings nor emotions, they came as I *listened with my body*; this is affect. Affect is non-passive openness and receptivity. Listening with the body creates affect. The sadness and aloneness I was feeling came in the form of a familiar and unspoken question, 'what do I do with this?' This question tends to shut down affect as we slip into the beginning of a story.

The two Sudanese drivers were locked into their knowledge of themselves, each other and their history of tribal and civil warfare. Although they had probably fled Sudan to escape the conflict, they had effectively recreated something of what they had tried to leave behind. The weariness I felt had less to do with their conflict, and more to do with how often and easily we trap ourselves within the emotionality of our tired stories.

By staying with affect, it becomes possible to avoid the suffering of our familiar stories. Even so, it is not possible to avoid the pain of affect when it is painful. While affect is not generally painful, it is often disrupting, and *it is always peaceful* since peace is not dependent on the absence of conflict. While affect can disrupt our balance, which is partly what makes it so valuable, it does not disturb the peace.

Empathy as defence against intimacy

Expressing sadness and a longing for peace might feel like care; however, taking part in a story in this way is a defence against affect and is very often also virtue signalling – if only to oneself. Conversely, by being open to affect I was free from empathy enabling me to avoid joining in. Knowledge of how to make the situation better is generally a defence against affect and uncertainty, had I joined in in this way I might have calmed the situation, but it would not have provided peace.

Emotions do not of themselves invite empathy, although emotionality is often taken as an invitation or opportunity for empathy. As a psychotherapist, it is often tempting to join in in this way since empathy is generally seen as attunement and therapeutic alliance. For example, the Sudanese observer might well have offered the hug thinking I needed comforting. He might have said to himself, 'I felt like *you* needed a hug', which, besides being a projection, would in all likelihood, have come from having interpreted my tears from within a personal, social or cultural story. I think the hug came from affect since he simply stretched out his arms and hugged me. The offer was not an expression of need, his or mine. It was not empathy, he did not have to imagine himself in my shoes and he was stood in them. I think the hug was a recognition of the unanticipated peace shared between two strangers as they melted away in the midst of a violent confrontation.

The hug was also a desire to embrace something other than the familiar story of tribal and civil war. It was surely harder for him to resist joining in, and yet unlike the two drivers he apparently had. By contrast, the tears of affect in our eyes were irresistible, he could not resist following a stranger down the street. The tears were unemotional, unfeeling, pre-personal, they were unknowing tears: *tears without a story*. I think this is what we both wanted to embrace.

To be clear, our connection existed before the altercation occurred and before we had met. It only became visible when we saw the tears in each other's eyes. As soon as this happened my weariness was gone allowing an underlying peace to brake out. Unintentionally and unknowingly, we had become peace-makers. With our openness to affect, we had co-created that which was not apparent. Peace cannot come from what is known.

Had he caught up with me, or had I caught up with him? The tears in my eyes were not mine, nor were they *not* not mine. We had mirrored one another. 'My' tears had apparently affected him, perhaps helping him not join in in the altercation, and perhaps him catching up with me had brought me back from the verge of going further into my own story. In affective encounters ownership and who-did-what-to-whom become meaningless.

Affect resonates on a different level than feelings and emotions. Feelings and emotions partly stem from a desire to connect with ourselves and others. Affect is the resonance of connection and a solvent for dissolving the illusion of separation. While some stories feel as though they bring people together and create a sense of belonging, it is more accurate to say that they *bind* people together. Whereas affect *loosens*, it does not bind, nor does it create belonging or connection, it *is* connection without knowing it, and without knowledge and intention, it uncovers peace, it does not create it. Affect only disturbs the peace by stirring it up within us.

Knowledge as a defence against affect

If knowledge were the greatest fairy tale ever told, we might wonder what kind of fairy tale psychotherapy is. When Freud retold Sophocles' Oedipus Rex as the Oedipus Complex, he intended to re-present the myth as scientific knowledge. Perhaps the best way to read Freud's Oedipus Complex is as a fairy tale in the manner of the Brothers Grimm. Although it has no fairies, there is an Oracle who can predict the future, and like the Brothers' Grimm, it is a bloody, cruel and violent story.

In what was ostensibly a story about one father's cruel brutality towards his son, Freud and Oedipus both set out to re-tell the story in their own separate ways. Freud's story seemed to be about the inevitability of incest, while Oedipus' was about an unavoidably disastrous reunion. In leaving the Oracle of Delphi behind, and in their eagerness to tell their own stories, Freud and Oedipus appeared to overlook, or perhaps miss the significance of the famous inscription 'Know thyself' carved in stone at the Temple of Apollo. Was this inscription intended as advice? Or perhaps as a commandment? Maybe it was a portentous warning to those who approach the Oracle? Or might it have been intended as a joke, an *in*-joke?

Certainly, the inscription can be read as ironic. After all, no amount of personal insight could have helped Oedipus discover his parentage. There is also a certain irony in seeking counsel when the message above the counsellor's door tells you to look for the answer within yourself. If it were intended as irony, for Oedipus at least, it would have been a cruel irony as we see his story quickly go from tragedy to tragicomedy.

While humour can be the most sophisticated form of defence, laughter is the supreme affect. The psychotherapist that is so defended that they are unable to laugh at themselves *and* their clients is not fit to work. For the psychotherapist perhaps, the greatest value in reading Oedipus Rex and Freud's Oedipus Complex comes from the affect they have upon the reader, and not from the knowledge they might glean. Perhaps their greatest value, and indeed the value of almost any psychotherapeutic theory, comes from seeing them as a parody of the pursuit of self-knowledge.

Freud wanted his followers to understand the point of the Oedipus Complex. This could be said of any psychotherapeutic theory: the point of the story is *to understand the point of the story*. Freud wanted his followers to understand psychoanalysis (as science) and then use (replicate) it in their work. This may be what distinguishes a theoretical story from a myth: theoretical stories are primarily instructional and intended for learning, whereas myths are told for affect.

Despite the affect Freud's ideas surely had upon himself, he did not want his followers to be so affected that they might deviate from the official narrative. Despite his own experience (and perhaps because of it), Freud effectively gave primacy to (his preferred) knowledge over affect.

For Freud's precursor, the philosopher and self-proclaimed *first psychologist* Friedrich Nietzsche, knowledge was only fit for camels. Nietzsche, who put affect before knowledge, asks, 'What is heavy? So asketh the load-bearing spirit; then kneeleth it down like the camel, and wanteth to be well laden' (Nietzsche, 1883/1969, p.54), part of his answer to this question takes the form of another question, '… to feed on the acorns and grass of knowledge, and for the sake of truth to suffer hunger of soul?' (Nietzsche, 1883/1969, p.54). Fortunately for the history of psychoanalysis and the future of psychotherapy, Freud's disciples were largely not content with being camels.

Nietzsche

In the often off-putting quasi-biblical language of *Thus Spake Zarathustra*, Nietzsche refers to the metamorphosis of the Camel. The Camel is a person with 'a load bearing spirit'; they are heavy, hard-working, unable to create, they accept society's values, they are beasts of burden, seeking only duty and that which is expected of them.

Bearing burden is the destiny of the Camel, their duty *is* their affect, it is also their morality. Any moral judgement regarding my affective response to the road rage incident is as unnecessary as it is irrelevant, since affect *is* itself moral. In other words, my tears were a moral response. Judging affect is a *secondary judgement* of what is a *primary judgement*. Secondary judgements are a form of appeal, they take place in our own *internal court of appeal*.

It is when we resist affect by entering into a story that we often find ourselves within the *internal court of appeal.* This is where prejudice, second-guessing and after-thought can be heard, whether guilty or not guilty, the process is mostly prejudicial, tiresome and predictable. The peculiar and farcical thing about the internal court of appeal is that judge and judged are one-in-the-same, and so *they are always equal to the task.*

In *Writings from the Late Notebooks*, Nietzsche remarks, '… moral evaluating is an *interpretation*, a way of interpreting. The interpretation itself is a *symptom* of particular physiological conditions, as well as a particular intellectual level among the ruling judgements. *Who interprets?* – Our affects' (Nietzsche, 2003, p.96). What stands out about this quote is that it is *our affects* that interpret, and that they are not a *what*; they are *who*. Nietzsche sees that *our affects are who we are.* Our moral valuations *are* our affects and they go to the heart of who we are. 'Morality is part of the theory of the affects: how closely do the affects approach the heart of existence?' (Nietzsche, 2003, p.60).

Nietzsche relates the following experience (which can also be read as a dream),

> One day recently at eleven o'clock in the morning a man suddenly collapsed right in front of me as if struck by lightning, and all the women in the vicinity screamed aloud; I myself raised him to his feet and attended to him until he had recovered his speech, during this time not a muscle of my face moved and

> I felt nothing, neither fear nor sympathy, but I did what needed doing and went coolly on my way. Suppose someone had told me the day before that tomorrow at eleven o'clock in the morning a man would fall down beside me in this fashion I would have suffered every kind of anticipatory torment, would have spent a sleepless night, and at the decisive moment instead of helping the man would perhaps have done what he did. For in the meantime all possible drives would have *had time* to imagine the experience and to comment on it. What then are our experiences? Much *more* that which we put into them than that which they already contain! Or must we go so far as to say: in themselves they contain nothing? To experience is to invent?
>
> (Nietzsche, 1881/1997, p.119)

Although Nietzsche could not anticipate the pre-personal affect of the man collapsing, he was aware that if he could have been told prior to it happening, he would have imagined any number of stories unfolding, and yet, like Oedipus, no amount of self-knowledge could have predicted his own behaviour.

Nietzsche's imagined response would have involved feelings and emotions making the encounter personal and social. Whereas his moral response, – *his affective response*, not only came before feeling and emotion, it precluded them. In this sense, psychotherapies that privilege emotional intelligence over affect are de-moralising. They are not so much morally equivocal – they are morally retarded.

Nietzsche suggests that advanced warning would have likely turned his experience into something of a crisis. How a person behaves in a crisis is often considered to be the best indication of their moral character. Affect does not ask us to go beyond our morals, it brings them into awareness. When Nietzsche said putting 'much more… into them [experiences] than that which they already contain!' (Nietzsche, 1881/1997, p.119), he is effectively describing the process of turning affect into a story: making some-thing out of no-thing. 'Or must we go so far as to say: in themselves they [experiences] contain nothing?' (Nietzsche, 1881/1997, p.119) to go so far as to say an experience contains nothing might also suggest that the 'substance' of nothing is affect? If this is so, are we then nothing?

How best to distrust yourself

Pierre Klossowski, in his book *The Vicious Circle*, which is primarily about Nietzsche's foremost idea *the eternal return of the same*, wrote, 'The more he [Nietzsche] listened to his body, the more he came to distrust the person the body supports' (Klossowski, 1997, p.24). With this in mind we might ask, 'how can we usefully distrust our own story-telling? And, 'how can we put this distrust to good use?' In whatever way we answer these questions, any answer probably entails no longer believing in ourselves or the belief that we know what we are doing.

The question of trust arises when we start listening *with* the body. The more we listen to the body (to affect), the more distrust we have of ourselves. It is notable that Klossowski does not transfer the placing of trust onto or into the body, – since we could not trust that which places the trust, it is as though trust itself is no longer trustworthy. Listening is better than trusting insofar as listening requires (and enables) the listener to remain open. Put another way, no one wants or needs a psychotherapist they trust if they have one that listens with their body, not only because it means they are open and unknowing, but also because such a listener can facilitate others to listen in this way.

A baby does not trust its body – it is a body, as it gets older it forgets this, and as its self and social consciousness grow it eventually imagines it has a self, and that this imagined self is somehow distinct from the body.

Affect's expansiveness sweeps away our sense of self which is not overwhelming since there is no one to overwhelm. After I had witnessed the altercation, and after the tears had washed me away, the feelings of sadness and aloneness arose as a story, as a defence against the expansiveness of affect. While feelings and emotions can be overwhelming, they are not expansive. However big the story, it will always keep things relatively small by anchoring us in the dramatic arc of *who we are*.

An alternative to truth

Since affect is not concerned with truth (although truth is perhaps a symptom of affect?), the value of affect may become premium in a so-called post-truth world. Appreciating the value of affect follows from an appreciation of how some of our oldest and most cherished values have now perished, and with them so too are the realities they once supported.

Had the two drivers witnessed the hug they could not have argued over the affect it had on either one of us, although they might – had we presented it as an alternative story to theirs. The moment affect gets taken up as a claim to truth it becomes a story, it is then something to argue over at the expense of its greatest value. The most valuable affect is laughter.

If we *are* affect, the *who* that interprets *is* affect, then we *as* affect are free of truth. This means when we are at our most moral, truth becomes irrelevant. It is not that morals are untruths, it is perhaps that they become impervious to truth and unable to resist laughter.

If affect is not a different kind of truth, it can become an alternative to truth. One of the most powerful things about working with affect, is its ability to make a psychotherapist more capable of laughter allowing them to become a stranger to the truth.

Creation myths

In one sense it all began for Freud with the Oedipus Complex which was once the corner-stone of psychoanalysis. Certainly much would come to be written about infant and early childhood development, and yet for Freud there was something about Oedipus Rex and his re-telling of it that held his attention.

By making *knowledge of good and evil* forbidden fruit, the writer(s) of the *Book of Genesis* did not exactly write a story about sex, though they did pave the way for the Church to write its own salacious creation story. In emphasising the sexual overtones of being 'beguiled' (Genesis 3:13), tempted, feeling 'naked' (Genesis 3:7), feeling shame, and 'eat[ing] of the fruit' (Genesis 3:3), what had been a story about the pleasure of curiosity and the danger of forbidden knowledge, became a sexualised and scandalising story about *knowledge as transgression.*

The Oedipus Complex and the story of The Garden of Eden are both morality tales about the transgression of eating forbidden fruit. In both the Oedipus Complex and the Church's interpretation of the third chapter of Genesis, the desire for knowledge became carnal desire. In both Freud's and Sophocles' interpretations of the life of Oedipus, wanting to know your mother does not simply mean finding out who she is. Had Freud and the Church been less obsessed with sex, they might have become more curious about what these stories had to say about the dangers of knowing.

Had the Church not had such a peculiar relationship with sex (is there such a thing as an un-peculiar relationship to sex?), we might wonder how differently the threat of curiosity would have been perceived. With Freud's shocking and scandalising story about how children sexually desire one parent, while harbouring potentially murderous intent towards the other, knowingly or unknowingly it was easy for Freud to distract (his and others) attention away from the threat of knowledge. By placing sexuality at the centre of a desire for knowledge, Freud and the Church drew our attention away from the thought that a desire for knowledge could simply be just that. If a desire for knowledge were just so, what might it be about knowledge that we need protecting from?

While God declared that Adam and Eve should not eat of the fruit of *the tree of knowledge of good and evil*, parents rarely make such a declaration about the taboo of incest. Parents tend to gently steer their child away, whereas God's prohibition may have also been an enticement, by creating such a tree, how could it not have been an accident *intended* to happen.

The incest taboo does not exist to be broken; nonetheless, parents and their children do desire each other. When it comes to incest, parents generally know about the 'good and evil' of incest while small children do not. They, like Adam and Eve, want something *of* their parents without necessarily knowing what it is, or what it might do for, or to them. Most parents succeed where God did not, despite and because of the child's efforts, most parents have enough boundaries without necessarily putting them into words. Whether or not God does things unintentionally is theologically open to question, but by forbidding them the fruit of knowledge, God (inadvertently?) created an object of desire. The parents' task is to frustrate incestuous desire (their own and their child's), and do it in such a way so as not to shame or quash the child's unknowing nascent desire. It is also important that parents do not try and work out their child's desire for them. In this sense, parents must make themselves available to be known in other desirable ways.

Wanting to 'know' a parent in the 'Biblical sense' and for that matter in the Oedipal sense turns knowing into a sexual act, but what about the dangers of the *act of knowing*? The Church is certainly way overdue for a revaluation of its relationship to sex, and therefore its peculiar and perverse relationship to knowledge. And for that matter, what of the *act of knowing* in psychotherapy?

Open curiosity and closed curiosity

Evidently Socrates' famous dictum that 'an unexamined life is not worth living' (Plato, 1966, p.38a) is false, there are innumerable worthwhile ways of living that do not require examination. Perhaps because Socrates is commonly thought of as the founder of western philosophy this misconception gets overlooked, and besides *no one wants truth to get in the way of a good story*. Ignoring the inconvenience of this, many psychotherapists have nonetheless taken this Socratic 'truth' and used it as a marketing strap-line.

'Know thyself' is another cherished and somewhat deceptive phrase taken from antiquity and adopted into the heart of psychotherapy. This apparently uncontentious little phrase reinforces what may well be the most pervasive iatrogenic disease in psychotherapy, namely a belief in self.

When God prohibited Adam and Eve from eating from the tree, they must have wondered what it had to do with them. Had they stayed with the affect of God's prohibition and the snake's beguilement, they might have seen God and the snake in a new light. They might have been able to see this prohibition as a reflection of the limitation of God. By taking God's prohibition personally, *by making it about themselves*, it was they that made themselves smaller, guilty and shameful. Their fall from grace had nothing to do with sin, their damnation was far worse, they had made themselves the centre of their world.

Had they obeyed God the result might have been much the same since obedience would merely have been a different version of the same story, albeit one based on fear. However, if instead they had experienced the (pre-personal) affect of God's words, they would likely have wondered what the prohibition said about God. Such curiosity would have been 'open curiosity': a curiosity that does not need to know. Whereas the curiosity they expressed was 'closed curiosity', a curiosity that needs to know.

Knowledge played an important role in the 'Fall of man' for both Adam and Eve, and also in the fall of Freud. Freud's fall was partly due to his insistence that psychoanalysis was science, and not a story or an experience. We can only wonder what might have happened to psychoanalysis had Freud seen that its greater value lay in its affect. Instead of embracing the affect his (and their) ideas undoubtedly had on his disciples, Freud preferred that psychoanalysts and their analysands stick to the story.

For Adam and Eve, the fruit of knowledge was the feeling of nakedness that accompanies self-consciousness. Feeling naked was evidently new to them, although they had vision, they had not 'seen' themselves before. 'Then the eyes of both [Adam and Eve] were opened and they knew they were naked…' (Genesis 3:7) when God called to them, Adam said, 'I heard the sound of thee in the garden, and I was afraid, because I was naked; and I hid myself' (Genesis 3:10). God could surely hear the shame in Adam's voice – his voice had broken, God would have instantly known that the taste of knowledge had brought with it a sense of self.

Those who seek a return to Eden do so because they see humanity as a corrupt and corrupting species. With their new sense of self, Adam and Eve effectively lost sight of their connection. When we no longer desire or are seduced by a sense of self we no longer seek to return to the Garden, for it then becomes clear that we had never left it.

The affect of dreaming and magical realism

Dreams are made of affect, Deleuze and Guattari's description of affect comes close to describing dream process, which is also 'a pre-personal intensity corresponding to the passage from one experiential state of the body to another' (Deleuze & Guattari, 1987, p. xvi).

Both affect and dreams are pre-personal. The body is experienced as affect, in this sense the body is pre-personal. The waking body and the sleeping body are the dream-body. Dreams are a manifestation of affect as it passes through the body.

While dreams are unique to the dreamer, they are nonetheless pre-personal in the peculiar and familiar way that we can experience our own body. A case in point is perhaps the most intimate and pre-personal relationship any person is ever likely to have. Those who have undergone fairly major surgery and met their surgeon not long before going under will likely testify to what quickly became a very intimate pre-personal relationship. Psychotherapy at its best tends to begin as a personal relationship, eventually, if permitted, it becomes a profoundly intimate and pre-personal relationship.

Dreamers do not tell a story as they dream, *dreams are not stories*, they are affect. It is only upon waking that the dreamer will likely turn a dream into a story. I could re-tell the road rage incident as a story, but that would change it by making it personal – about me, or social – as a commentary about modern life or civil war. To illustrate the distinction, I shared my experience of the road rage incident with someone I work with, as I did so it was as though I were recalling a dream. The affect it had on them was similar to my own, they also had tears in their eyes.

Sharing this experience with my client had an unanticipated affect on me, I too had tears, it was no less affecting now than it had been when I witnessed the altercation. It was as if *they* were sharing the experience with me, it had become as much theirs as it was mine. This was also reflected in what happened with the Sudanese man: it was not clear whether he had 'caught' up with me, or I with him.

Had I told the experience as a story I suspect my client would have asked how I was feeling. They did not need to, they had experienced the immediacy of affect themselves. As a story it would have conveyed feelings and emotions, to which my client would likely have responded with empathy which would have prevented the experience from becoming theirs. Despite appearances, empathy is all too often a defence against affect and intimacy.

The experience now belonged as much to my client, as it did to myself and the Sudanese man. An experience belongs to those affected by it. It struck me that telling a story is a form of privatisation, – a capitalist enterprise, whereas shared affect is a sort of 'multiplication miracle'. The pre-personal nature of affect prevents exclusive ownership, although my client and the Sudanese man had never met, they were now as connected to each other as I was to either of them. Affect belongs to no one, it can only be said to belong to anyone in the way that the vibration of a violin string belongs to the violin. In this sense, the affect we experience in or on 'our' body belongs to no one. And insofar as bodies *are* affect, they too belong to no-one.

The experience of the altercation and the hug, and of sharing it with my client, was not dream-like, we *were* dreaming. Although I do not know if this is how they experienced it, we were affectively lucid dreaming while awake. This is not lucid dreaming in the conventional sense. Lucidity is not only when the sleeping dreamer becomes aware they are dreaming, it is also when the dreamer becomes aware that they are always dreaming, in other words, what is thought to be waking up out of a dream is merely the transition from sleeping to waking. Affective lucidity is also the dreamer's realisation that they are no more the person they identify with in the dream than they are the person asleep in bed having the dream, and further still, nor are they the person who records the dream when they awake.

There are different ways to help yourself stay with the lucidity of affect. Asking yourself several times a day, 'am I dreaming?' is a good way to bring attention to affect as it can interrupt any story you are inhabiting, or about to. Since stories require narration, thinking without words can help inhibit narrating stories in your thoughts, making it easier to stay with affect. Noticing how you speak in your dreams can be a useful guide for how to speak with affect. Words spoken and thought in dreams tend to be few, sentences are often short, simple, and to the point. They do not always make sense since words in dreams tend to convey affect rather than being a form of communication.

We do not expect to see cause and effect in dreams, and so looking for it is a quick and reliable way out of lucidity. When lucid, we are less likely to question the uncanny or apparently magical. For example, when flying in a dream you might immediately wake up and then think it was the impossibility of flight that awoke you. This is unlikely since the unexpected and magical are common in dreams – flying is normal, what often wakes a person up out of a 'flying dream' is the dreamer attempting to frame it within cause and effect in order to know how to fly.

One aspect of the genius of the writer Gabriel García Márquez's *One Hundred Years of Solitude* is how the magical seems normal or 'real', and the everyday appears strange and uncanny. Needless to say, with the 'magical realism' of his writing, cause and effect, and the passage of time do not apply in any conventional sense, and not unlike a dreamer, the reader soon stops looking for, and expecting to find them.

Márquez's characters appear to be driven and animated by affect, typically they do not have richly drawn internal lives, and yet despite – and more likely because of this, they are deeply affecting. Through his alchemical writing style Márquez manages to dissolve the (imagined) dichotomy between magic and reality distilling them into affect. The psychotherapist who, like Márquez, works creatively with affect will become a magical realist.

Conclusion

Putting affect into words entails borrowing from the language of feeling and emotion. Borrowed language almost inevitably returns home taking the experience with it. Although using the language of feeling and emotion to describe affect is unavoidable, it tends to lead to a confusion and conflation of what are distinctly different phenomena.

Affect as truth

Affect does not redefine or rehabilitate truth. If affect is any kind of truth at all, it is neither correspondent nor propositional. Affect has no equivalence and it proposes nothing. Affective truth is the body *as* affect, as 'it' passes through. If it were a kind of truth it would be truth *as* process, not content, and so the truth of a piece of writing resides, – as exemplified by Nietzsche, in the affect of its style upon the reader.

It should be noted that if truth is a quality of affect, or vice versa, truth would be one of affect's least valuable qualities.

For Nietzsche, the affect of truth is laughter, 'And we should call every truth false which was not accompanied by at least one laugh' (Nietzsche, 1883/1969, p.228). If laughter is the ultimate expression of truth, and the best way to discern it, laughter has still greater value. The highest value of laughter comes as an affirmation of life.

Affect as morality

Affective morality does not permit us the claim of *being* moral or congruent. They are not (cannot) be the aim of a psychotherapy of affect. Instead morality and congruence are symptoms of affect. Any student of psychotherapy reading this will likely recognise the mantra, *process over content*. For traditional psychotherapy process over content is primarily about learning the priority of focus. For a psychotherapy of affect, it is also ethical.

The morality of affect is pre-personally congruent which means that it is unlikely to feel congruent according to a sense of self, if there is one. The greater a person's sense of self, the more transgressive affect will likely feel. Since the morality of affect is incidental, the ethics of a psychotherapist of affect will depend upon the openness of their curiosity.

A psychotherapy of affect

Beyond Good and Evil was the title of one of Nietzsche's most famous works, it does not refer to a destination, it is perspectival. Beyond is not a temporal progression or regression: there is no *going* beyond either forward into the future, or back into the past. It is the perspective of going nowhere and having no purpose.

The psychotherapy of affect is purposeless, it is able to go nowhere partly because it is beyond good and evil. It does not seek to return or go beyond, it accepts there is nowhere to go and no need to go there. By becoming self-conscious of guilt and shame, Adam and Eve discovered what it means *to be*, and with it they found a sense of purpose based on no longer feeling whole. It was perhaps inevitable that religions and indeed psychotherapies would root themselves in the belief of self, guilt, shame, and good and evil.

With their nascent self-consciousness, Adam and Eve felt guilt and shame for the first time, and with it they created separation and a need for connection with themselves and each other. These self-created feelings led to the original sin: they had placed themselves at the centre of the world. By contrast a psychotherapy of affect is *de-centring*, any sense of self is dispersed, it is as though we *move beyond ourselves*, except, since there is no one to move and nowhere to go, it is affect that flows, moving *through* bodies, not between them.

In this way, an affective sense of self is similar to the lucid dreamer's sense of self. The 'dream self' is both dispersive and inclusive; it includes all aspects of the dream as it disperses everywhere, into nothing and nowhere. Affect does not seek connection, it eradicates the desire for it and the illusion of separateness that created the desire.

Insofar as there is no 'affective self', *there is no affect*, – there is only a sense of them. Nonetheless, since traditional psychotherapy will continue to help people find themselves, it will fall to the psychotherapy of affect to help people lose themselves.

References

Deleuze, G and Guattari, F (1980/1987) *A Thousand Plateaus: Capitalism and Schizophrenia,* Vol. 2. trans. B. Massumi. Minneapolis and London: University of Minnesota Press.

Klossowski, P (1969/1997) *Nietzsche and the Vicious Circle,* trans. D. W. Smith. London: The Athlone Press.

Nietzsche, F (1881/1997) *Daybreak,* trans. R. J. Hollingdale. Cambridge: Cambridge University Press.

Nietzsche, F (1883/1969) *Thus Spake Zarathustra: A Book for All and None,* trans. R. J. Hollingdale. London: Penguin.

Nietzsche, F (1886/1979) *Beyond Good and Evil: Prelude to a Philosophy of the Future,* trans. R. J. Hollingdale. London: Penguin.

Nietzsche, F (2003) *Writings from the Late Notebooks,* trans. K. Sturge. Cambridge: Cambridge University Press.

Plato, (1966) *Plato in Twelve Volumes*, Vol. 1, trans. H. N. Fowler. Cambridge: Harvard University Press.

Chapter 8

Taking orders from the night

Manu Bazzano

To David Armstrong (1934-2026), Social Dreaming pioneer

The sleep of reason?

Taking orders from the night implies being open to dreams – the main topic of this investigation. It also suggests becoming receptive to what emerges when, unable to sleep, one succeeds in giving up the injunction to fall asleep and remain instead alert and responsive to images, memories, thoughts, and feelings emerging in the dark. Why do these phenomena feel at once purer and harsher at night? In my case at present, being awake at night is partly due to the medication I have been taking for some time, but there may be other reasons too that are hard to fathom. This may sound strange, but at times it feels as if I am attending to presences sitting at the foot of the bed. In their more nightmarish manifestations, they remind me of Goya's paintings, the hideous merging with sullenness and humour.

Whether in a dream or lying awake in the dark, milder appearances may bring insights outside the linear train of reason. Some visitations perturb reason, and if reason is not ousted, it will come out stronger and better placed in the psychical landscape. For what is reason but another affect?

The heart has its reasons that reason knows nothing of, in the words of Pascal, echoed in Redon's painting of 1887 where a naked man stands on a balcony with his right hand reaching inside a slit in his chest to feel his heart. In Failla's short story *Pascal's Night of Fire,* the 31-year-old Blaise Pascal has a terrifying and transformative encounter with his faceless double during a sleepless night on November 23, 1654. The night encounter will bring about a *conversion*, a change of heart (Failla, 2016).

The night is *Lilah*, dark beauty, the unexplainable, what we cannot see, and infinite carpet of stars, no landing strip or visible landmarks (Sandman, 1997). Historically, artists and poets approached this domain with respect. I wish the same could be said for psychotherapists.

*

DOI: 10.4324/9781003669906-9

> Walking alongside a cliff on the North Devon coast, I hear people's cries of awe, of wonder and terror from the sea down below. I see a whale, rising up, I too feel awe and terror. I wake up feeling joyful. When I recount the dream at the matrix a week later, someone suggests wailing, and in the associations that follow the tears of joy become the tears for Ariadne's lost thread. Will we be lost in the labyrinth after slaying the Minotaur? Is love the lost thread? Have we misplaced the rituals and invocations that could conjure up the thread?

*

A dream is an affect in visual garment. It belongs to the unsung domain of the *soul*, understood with the ancient Greeks as *ψυχῆ*, psyche, an expansive sphere that goes well beyond the atomized, impoverished notion of the individual soul inherited by the prevailing interpretations of religious texts. The soul remains forever "undiscovered, though explored forever to a depth beyond description" (Heraclitus, 2001, p. 45, translation modified). Even when we are "submerged in sleep [it] is hard at work and helps make something of the world" (Heraclitus, 2001, p. 57). Not only does soul comprises the whole universe – *anima mundi*, the soul of the world and the world ensouled, in Hillman's felicitous turn of phrase (1998). Its work takes place imperceptibly, unheeded, and unperturbed by cognitive directives and manipulations.

Mainstream therapy promotes self-care, a notion that is constitutive of neoliberal modes of living, an insipid reflection of the *care of self* championed by ancient Greek philosophy. It worships a reductive notion of the self, of its emblems, projects, and fears, of its greed and vanity. It professes to shield it from the numerous *triggers* (an obligatory term in current discourse) that may affect, challenge, and God forbid, *transform* our default and often blinkered worldview. It cares for an atomized, confined view of what constitutes individuality to which it then confusedly appends the notion of soul. This error is not new; it harks back to Cartesianism, a mode of thought fashionably berated in academia but unquestioned in its core notion of the *cogito* and its enmeshment with the atomized soul of conventional theistic beliefs.

In some cases, mainstream therapy annexes *spirit* to a reductive self-construct. The result is the fashioning of approaches that feature insights and practices from spiritual traditions. All well and good but for one crucial factor: spirit *bypasses* soul entirely. It bypasses ambivalence, ambiguity, and fruitful uncertainty. It bypasses nuance. It ignores a vast liminal sphere that is pregnant with intimations, reverberations, and visitations. The move from self to spirit is a jolt: I was riding a bicycle through uneven terrain; now I suddenly find myself on an aeroplane, looking down on that very same terrain.

Too much concern with the self and its endless dramas – its aversions, cravings, and perpetual wish for specialness and validation – turns psychotherapeutic investigation into a tangled, uninspiring mess. The flight to spirit may add spaciousness, a welcome if illusive bird's eye view on our struggles before we go back to our familiar narratives. The mixture of rationality and mysticism that is the product of this repetitive, unsatisfactory undertaking cannot in good faith be called psychotherapy, for psychotherapy is cure of the *psyche*, or a type of cure that necessitates an investigation of the soul.

An intermediate terrain

As *affects* in visual attire, dreams cannot be mechanically demoted to oracular visitations, to symptoms of frustrated drives or the labyrinthine aftermath of physiological needs. They do not fit with narrow notions of the body and subjectivity, or with equally narrow notions of spirit. They belong to an *intermediate* terrain. They belong to the ambiguous realm of soul or *psyche*. Ambiguity implies that the dream cannot be made to serve the bolstering of consciousness in relation to living. It is wrong – *exegetically insulting* (Hillman, 1979) – to drill a dream in order to feed our scheming and strategizing. It is inadequate as well as deceptive. Dreams' connection with soul implies deep connection with our death. *To deceive a dream is to deceive our own death.*

Working with dreams, especially in groups, helps us realize the futility of our attempts at gaining mastery over the life of the psyche. There is more: genuine proximity with a dream will confuse our sense of waking-life reality in interesting ways. The Taoist sage Chuang-Tzu dreamt he was a butterfly and woke up genuinely perplexed as to whether he was a butterfly now dreaming of being Chuang-Tzu.

Greater intimacy with the domain of affect – whether through dreamwork, Zen practice, Butoh, Rhizomatics, and other disciplines/traditions that are not sold to the hubris of our age – often implies developing a greater sense of perplexity. This can take different hues: from a sense of wonder that is close to the aesthetic/artistic perspective to an unsettling doubt about the existence of what we call reality, including the reality of the self.

The Korean Zen tradition typifies perplexity succinctly with the koan "What is this?". As with all koans, this is a far-reaching existential question with transformative potential. When we sincerely ask that question from the core of our being, the implied assertion we make is, *I don't know*. (Batchelor, 2019). Asking *What is this?* – in relation to the totality of this moment, life-and-death streaming through me, the sound of a passing train, grey clouds and a patch of blue on the horizon, this heart beating, a door being shut next door – may awake a sense of perplexity that is generative rather than merely confusing.

In Tolstoy's *Anna Karenina*, Levin (a character as central as Karenina and partly drawn on the author himself) is overwhelmed with joy when he realizes that the miracles he was after through abstract values and ideals were there all along within the folds of everyday existence. What greater miracles can there be? When approached with humility, dreams potentially obfuscate the certainties of waking life, which may lead to greater appreciation of the inherently enigmatic nature of existence. This is a first important step. Were we to stop here, however, we'd risk attributing to the dreamworld a literal oracular power. We would come close to the superstitious mumbo-jumbo of the New Age.

The second step happens through free association. The dream content and imagery are problematized, expanded, through a process of actively resisting facile interpretations, be it through anagogic leaps or symbolization.

The dream rhizome

Commenting on Prospero's famous line *We are such stuff as dreams are made on*, the psychoanalyst Gordon Lawrence (2018) perceived a third implication alongside the two more obvious ones. It is not merely that life is a dream and that we dream. We too are a dream, a dream that dreams. This sounds intriguing if a little bit disturbing in emphasizing the ephemerality of our existence and perhaps conveying, in the words of Miguel de Unamuno (2005), a tragic sense of life.

What *are* dreams? Are they individual, i.e., do they belong to a personal psyche? Can they be owned (as in "last night I *had* a dream")? For one thing, the uncanny (*unheimlich*, unhoused) visual metaphors they present us with provide a printout of our "connection or disconnection with the world about us". (Ullman, 1975, p. 9). Are dreams *visitations*, the irruption of otherness in the confines of our self? Could they signal the existence of a terrain that is wider than our private domain? Crucially, is the conscious mind adequate in shedding light on a dream? Even the term "shedding light" feels ineffective, betraying an invasive stance, taking the forensic light of reason into the night realm. Even if we decide to see dreams as a natural response to biological processes, the conscious mind will still be incapable of tracing their complexities. We need instead a methodology that is "congruent with unconscious processes, [one that] does not betray them" and does not hide behind "reductionist ratiocination" (Ullman, 1975, p. 9).

The methodology in question may be defined as blind knowledge, akin to what Freud was trying to convey to Salomé, a notion found in the writing of Gabriel Marcel (1965) and Bion (1992). It is also similar to what the Zen tradition refers to as five degrees of "blindness" or unknowing (Bazzano, 2016).

To Gordon Lawrence we owe the creation in 1982 of *social dreaming*, a practice of communal dreaming that unequivocally affirms that we would to better at discarding our ingrained belief that dreams belong to the individual.

The collective frame of social dreaming, working as it does via free association (rather than interpretation) and the construction of a reservoir of images and affective resonances, activates a twofold shift: from the individual to the collective and from the collective to the dreams themselves. The second shift implies that *we are not doing group work* but engaging with the more direct, *affect-driven* activity of oneiromancy or dreamwork. As with affect therapy, which focuses directly on the neutral, autonomous current of affect traversing the room and the bodymind of the individual client/patient, so with this mode of dreamwork: the focus is on the dreams themselves.

Dreams may well be the royal way to the unconscious, but the unconscious is a lot more than repressed psychic material relating to the individual who dreams. To embark on this exploration, we need a more expansive notion of the unconscious. Think of Proust, in whose writings every emotion and sensation is multiplied, reverberating ad infinitum, shepherding us into an intricate sequence of experiences and ephemeralities springing from memory and imagination. Think of Bergson (2011) through Deleuze (1991). Think of the *virtual*, the mist of virtual images encircling actuality and facticity, hinting at a pre-individual, pre-human province – not mere potentiality, but the virtual as fully real.

Dreamwork conceived in this way is useful in getting an immediate sense of what *affect therapy* (Bazzano, forthcoming) is about. It radically differs from the conventional way of understanding and working with dreams. It does so in several ways, including:

- The dream is at the centre, not the dreamer.
- There is no elucidation of the past, but an inquiry geared towards the future.
- No dramatization of personal biography but instead an emphasis, after Unamuno, of the tragic nature of existence.
- Not Oedipus, but the Sphinx.
- Not egocentric but sociocentric.
- Not overly concerned with the finite dimension but keen to explore the infinite dimension.
- Not resorting to Jungian/Platonist archetypes in order to "explain" dreams but relying entirely on free association, phenomenological inquiry, and a broadly Deleuzian paradigm.

Matrix and rhizome

The style of communal dreaming presented here is inspired by and greatly indebted to Gordon Lawrence's social dreaming and the "matrix", the latter term defining both a *form* and a *process* as specified in his last book:

> As a form, [the matrix] is a configuration of people that provides a unique space, or 'container' for thinking out of the content of dreams to consider and discover their hidden, elusive/infinite meaning. As a process, the matrix is the system or web of emotions and thinking that is present in every social relationship, but for the most part unattended and not acknowledged. It can be thought of as mirroring while awake, the infinite, unconscious processes in waking life that give rise to dreaming when asleep.
>
> (Lawrence, 2005, pp. 14–15)

Personally, I have learned and continue to learn greatly as a participant in a particular matrix. I have also experimented with it when hosting communal dreaming as part of the events I facilitate. While feeling respectful of and indebted to the form and process of the matrix, I confess to some resistance in calling it matrix. The etymology suggests the breeding womb of the mother; it hints at an origin, a ground from which dreams and associations allegedly stem. This does not quite align with my own experience. Dreams in the communal dreaming experience, even the first dream that kicks off the process, are already embedded in a composite net of connections. We are, so to speak always starting in the middle. The same is true for subsequent dreams and for the associations that follow. The term I use instead of matrix is, after Deleuze, *rhizome*, and refers to my experimentations with communal dreaming as *Dream Rhizome*.

The rhizome

A rhizome is a circular, horizontal structure of ramifications consisting of underground stems – e.g., bulbs and tubers. In contrast to roots, a rhizome does not grow via binary splits. *Rhizomatics* (the image in psychology and philosophy that I am using here in relation to communal dreamwork) is at variance with the prevailing metaphors of the tree and the root – as well as the matrix and/or the womb – conventionally applied to describe the world, experience, and life. The tree metaphor depicts linear, developing, structured systems. Linearity, development, and structure as conceived within this metaphor are ubiquitous in current notions of psychological "growth", whether in relation to trauma studies or more generally in human development. The root metaphor relies on the notion of unity; the difference is that unity here is either concealed or dormant. The unconscious (when understood phylogenetically as the "ground of being") must be made conscious, the past understood and redeemed or nostalgically retrieved; or: the latent must be actualized, the "authentic" come to the fore. These various images and metaphors are integral to the philosophical and psychotherapeutic tradition. What Lawrence's social dreaming instigates, however, belongs to a different mode of inquiry which I have for some time now labelled counter-traditional. As it often happens with innovators, they themselves are not fully aware of what they have creatively unleashed. And it is in that spirit that I feel confident in using, and working with the rhizome metaphor.

The rhizome is an underground yet evident network of several branching roots and shoots, with no central axis, no point of origin, and no pre-established direction of growth – a multiplying, to some degree chaotic, and differentiated system of growth. It is grounded on associations, divergencies, and multiplicities.

Here is how Deleuze and Guattari put it (2013, pp. 20–21):

> Unlike trees or their roots, the rhizome connects any point to any other point, and its traits are not necessarily linked to traits of the same nature; it brings into play very different regimes of signs, and even nonsign states. The rhizome is reducible neither to the One nor the multiple. It is not the One that becomes Two or even directly three, four, five, etc. It is not a multiple derived from the One, or

> to which One is added (n + 1). It is composed not of units but of dimensions, or rather directions in motion. It has neither beginning nor end, but always a middle (milieu) from which it grows and which it overspills.

Dreams and the associations that shadow them are forms that *condense* (as with the German term for poetry *Gedichte* with its root in *dicht* = condensed) a composite array of emotional tendencies and intensities. A "meaning" that may emerge in the process is not a given deduced by cognitive interpretation but is more akin to *negative capability* – what John Keats described in a letter dated 21 December 1817 to his brothers Tom and George as the ability, found in Shakespeare, "of being in uncertainties, Mysteries, doubts, without any irritable reaching after fact & reason" (Keats, 2009). An ability to sustain lived uncertainty is crucial at two levels, one *particular* and the other *expansive*.

At the particular level, we need to rethink *partial objects* (Deleuze and Guattari, 2013) and no longer relegate them to the margins or explain them away as stages and/or offshoots in a developmental trajectory. Their potential menace and explosive, disruptive – at heart *political* – nature must be taken fully into account away from reactive attempts towards normalization, integration, and wholeness.

At the expansive level, one would need to think of affects as no longer akin to individual emotions and feelings. Feelings are personal and biographical; emotions are social; affects are pre-personal. *Affect is not a personal feeling* but a body experience of intensity taking place before language and conscious thought. One could think of affects as beings in themselves traversing the subject's bodymind and exceeding it. Or, even better as nonhuman becomings traversing the human.

Melanie Klein's discovery of partial objects was momentous. Less compelling was her insistence to unify and integrate them, based on the view that they constitute the negative source of the paranoid-schizoid position. Partial objects don't need unification in relation to a pre-determined whole, a view that is the underlying dogma in contemporary trauma narratives. Unification between the parts occurs not via the essentially repressive attempts at unification but through *desire*, understood not as craving and/or reactivity born of lack but as an active force devoid of either object or subject, a force that is able to create reality:

> If desire produces, its product is real. If desire is productive, it can be productive only in the real world and can produce reality.
>
> (Deleuze and Guattari, 1977, p. 26)

If a dream is an affect in visual attire, affect may be in turn understood as the *unthought known*, a feeling or cluster of feelings traversing and inhabiting us before becoming thought by way of a composite process of approximation, association and, partly, repression.

What Spinoza conceived of as the main affects – pleasure, pain, and desire – have one thing in common: they occur in activity. Aiding and increasing the power of action in the body indicates the coming into play of *active* forces. Restraining, diminishing that same power is on the other hand the work of *reactive* forces. When applied to the dream, the deceptively simple practice of free association may be seen as a good instance of active forces at play. Accosting the dream in its own terms, attuning oneself with humility to the dream's idiom while allowing for an open proliferation of images, affects, and thoughts to come through is entirely different from attempting to explain the dream through archetypal categorization, symbolization, and so forth.

Symmetry

Dream logic is a logic of *symmetry*, freely sidestepping the functional divisions characteristic of waking life. The Chilean psychoanalyst Matte-Blanco (1975, 1999) rewrites the unconscious from the viewpoint of mathematical set theory, a perspective which has invited intriguing comparisons with the fiction of Borges, a writer known for his compelling use of literary hints, of symmetry, for the exchangeability of reader, author, and fictional character and for the dissolution of chronology (Priel, 1994).

Symmetry and asymmetry, clarity, and "blindness", going in the dark without a light to find the songs and blossoms emerging from the dark: these allegories may also be rendered, as it happens in the Zen tradition, in terms of light and darkness. *Within light there is darkness*, we chant on *sesshins* (zen retreats), *but do not try to understand that darkness. Within darkness there is light, but do not look for that light* (Zen Mountain Monastery, Internet file). These notions are on one level ungraspable – unless the mind slows down in silent contemplation, surrendering its dependency on binary vision – unless we approach the dream momentarily suspending our habitual acquisitive logic.

Bibliography

Armstrong, D. (2018) 'Thinking Aloud: Contributions to Three Dialogues'. In W. G. Lawrence (2018), *Social Dreaming at Work*. Abingdon: Routledge, pp. 91–106.
Batchelor, S. (2019) *What Is This? Ancient Questions for Modern Minds*. New York: Tuwhiri Project Ltd.
Bazzano, M. (2016) 'Planting an Oak in a Flowerpot'. in R. Chisholm, and J. Harrison, (Eds) *The Wisdom of Not-Knowing*. Axminster: Triarchy Press, pp. 83–92.
Bazzano, M. (forthcoming) *Affect Therapy: A Manifesto*. Unpublished manuscript.
Bergson, H. (2011) *Matter and Memory*. Santa Fe, NM: Martino Fine Books.
Bion, W. R. (1992) *Cogitations*. London: Karnac Books.
Deleuze, G. (1991) *Bergsonism*. New York: Zone Books.
Deleuze, G. and Guattari, F. (1977) *Anti-Oedipus: Capitalism and Schizophrenia*. New York: Penguin Classics.
Deleuze, G. and Guattari, F. (2013) *A Thousand Plateaux*. London: Bloomsbury Academic.
Failla, S. G. (2016) 'Tears of Joy: Pascal's Night of Fire'. in M. Bazzano, and J. Webb, (Eds) *Therapy and the Counter-tradition: the Edge of Philosophy*. Abingdon: Routledge, pp. 58–64.

Freud, S, Letter to Lou Andreas-Salome, May 26, 1916, *The International Psycho-Analytical Library*, 89: 43 https://pep-web.org/browse/document/ipl.089.0045a, retrieved 23 June 22.

Heraclitus (2001) *Fragments*. Translated by Brooks Haxton, with an introduction by James Hillman. London: Penguin.

Hillman, J. (1979) *The Dream and the Underworld.* New York: Harper Perennial.

Hillman, J. (1998) *The Thought of the Heart and the Soul of the World.* Thompson, CT: Spring Publications.

Keats, J. (2009) Selection from Keath's Letters, *Poetry Foundation*, https://www.poetryfoundation.org/articles/69384/selections-from-keatss-letters accessed 23 Mar. 25

Lawrence, G. W. (2005) *An Introduction to Social Dreaming*. London: Karnac.

Lawrence, G. W. (2018) *Social Dreaming at Work*. Abingdon, OX: Routledge.

Matte-Blanco, I. (1975) *The Unconscious as Infinite Sets: An Essay in Bi-Logic*. London: Duckworth.

Matte-Blanco, I. (1999) *Thinking, Feeling, and Being: Clinical Reflections on the Fundamental Antinomy of Human Beings and the World*. London and New York: Routledge.

Marcel, G. (1965) *Being and Having: An Existential Diary*. New York: Joanna Cotler Books.

Priel, B. (1994) 'Symmetry: Matte-Blanco's Theory and Borges's Fiction'. *International Journal of Psychoanalysis*, August: 75 (Pt 4), pp. 815–823.

Salomé, L. (2001) *Nietzsche*, trans S. Mandel. Champaign, IL: University of Illinois Press.

Sandman, M. (1997) Lilah, a song from Morphine's album *Like swimming.* New York: Rykodisc.

Tolstoy, L. (2003) *Anna Karenina, (Part 8 Chapter 12)*. London: Penguin.

Ullman, M. (1975) 'The Transformation Process in Dreams'. New York: *The American Academy of Psychoanalysis*, 19 (2), pp. 8–10.

Ulman, M. (1981) 'Psi Communication through Dream Sharing'. *Parapsychological Review*, 12 (2), pp. 1.

De Unamuno, M. (2005) *Tragic Sense of Life*. New York: Cosimo Classics.

Chapter 9

Life as will to nothingness

Nihilism and affect in Nietzsche's third essay of the Genealogy of Morals

Margarita Karkagianni

The role of affect and affectivity in Nietzsche's *Genealogy of Morals* is an ongoing and recurring topic both in recent and earlier studies. Genealogy in the sense that it assumes in Nietzsche necessitates an understanding of affect and affectivity. Starting with Max Scheler's critique of Nietzsche's concept of *ressentiment* as the distinctive characteristic of Christianity (Scheler, 1975) up to the most recent attempts to read the *Genealogy of Morals* as a series of psychological studies where affective states, and particularly *ressentiment* appears to condition not only the birth of Christianity and its persistence in modern culture, but also the self-undermining of the person who endorses these ideals (Reginster, 2021), an examination of affect and affectivity becomes crucial for understanding Nietzsche's *genealogical* thought.

The following inquiry examines the role of affect in the third essay of the *Genealogy of Morals* in relation to the problem of life and the radical denial of life embodied in the ascetic ideal. The underlying question motivating this study is whether, in Nietzsche's treatment of the ascetic ideal and its role within life itself, the possibility arises to think affect beyond human psychology; whether indeed there is a type of affectivity that pertains to life per se. The first part of the chapter examines the relationship between the will to nothingness and the *nihil* of the will, in an attempt to bring forth the unique character of Nietzsche's treatment of the problem of nihilism in the third essay of the *Genealogy* as well as his account of the relationship between nihilism and the problem of life. The second part investigates the meaning(s) of the ascetic ideal for art and philosophy, the persistence of the ascetic ideal in modernity – i.e., philosophy's "will to truth" – the question of the possibility of philosophy today and finally the role of the life-denying principle within life itself. The third part examines the use of affect by the ascetic priest in his endeavour to save the human will from extinction and the two types of affectivity that determine the distinction between the strong and the weak, or, more generally, the ascending and declining movements within life itself.

The will to nothingness and the *nihil* of the will

One of the most remarkable aspects of Nietzsche's theory of the will is its intimate relation to affect. Even before the development of the theory of the will

DOI: 10.4324/9781003669906-10

to power, where the will is defined primarily as an affect – i.e., *the affect of command* – Nietzsche dissects the belief in "free will" in the terms that compose it; notably, the *feeling of power*, that accompanies the mastering and command of the resisting "underwills," and inversely, the affect of obedience from the perspective of those resisting wills that succumb to the domineering will (Nietzsche, 1966, pp.26–27). This close connection between will and affect is further developed and underlined in the posthumous notes, subsequently published as *The Will to Power.* Very significant in this respect is Nietzsche's critique of the mechanistic interpretation of the world in note 635 of the aforementioned work. Here Nietzsche concludes that if we eliminate from the mechanistic theory these elements that are borrowed from the metaphysical interpretation of nature – i.e., the concept of number, the concept of the "thing" and the belief in the unity of the ego that underlies it, the notions of activity and motion, understood as the movement between inert atoms – we are left only with "dynamic quanta, in a relation of tension to all other dynamic quanta" (Nietzsche, 1968, §635, p.339). As Deleuze observes, all dynamic quanta being related to all other dynamic quanta, "the relationship between forces in each case is determined to the extent that each force is *affected* by other, inferior or superior, forces. It follows that will to power is manifested as a capacity for being affected" (Deleuze, 1996, p.62). Stated more strongly, "the will to power not a being, not a becoming, but a *pathos* – the most elemental fact from which a becoming and effecting first emerge" (Nietzsche, 1968, § 635, p.339).

In light of the above, the problem that Nietzsche ventures to examine in the third essay of the *Genealogy of Morals* is bound to appear doubly enigmatic. It is well known that the last essay of the *Genealogy* is devoted to the problem of the meaning of the ascetic ideal. Yet, already from the start it becomes evident that the problem of the meaning of the ascetic ideal is intimately related with the problem of the human will. Thus, after a brief reference to the different senses of the ascetic ideal for artists, philosophers, the majority of mortals, and finally, priests, Nietzsche writes:

> *That* the ascetic ideal has meant so many things to man, however, is an expression of the basic fact of the human will, its *horror vacui: it needs a goal* – and it will rather will *nothingness* than *not* will.
>
> (Nietzsche, 1989, III, §1, p.97)

This dilemma that manifests itself at the heart of the human will addresses yet another problem that is foundational to the other two: nihilism. The problem of nihilism is addressed here in two decisive ways: in terms of the will that *wills nothingness* and the will which is swallowed by nothingness; that is, the will which is self-annihilated through the total absence of aim. In this sense, the will selects the "nothing" as its aim in order to evade the greatest danger – its self-annihilation.

Often, however, the will that wills nothingness and the will which is led to its self-annihilation are interpreted as two moments of the same will. What seems to preside in both is the *affect towards death.*

Karl Löwith (1997) explores precisely this view of "present-day" nihilism. He considers modern nihilism as an interim stage between the collapse of the Christian ideals and Nietzsche's vision of the counter-ideal: the Dionysian worldview with its affirmative stance towards life. The liberation of the will from the "Thou shalt" of Christian religion and morality, at first, presents itself as sickness – i.e., the realization that the world as such has no intrinsic value or meaning, hence the feeling that everything is "in vain"—and then, as "freedom towards death" (pp.47–48). For Löwith, these two stages demarcate the transition from passive to active nihilism. The latter strengthens the will to the extent that through this active will of destruction, even of self-destruction, the will recovers its resoluteness – the freedom to decide over itself and its fate; the liberation of the person, who has regained the capacity to will for him/herself to the extent that he/she can also decide over his/her own death:

> As long as the Christian gravity prevailed, man was held firmly into existence. One thought one knew why one is there at all, for the sake of what goals. The suffering of being-there was interpreted; the monstruous emptiness, the "horror vacui" seemed to be filled; "the door to suicidal nihilism was closed."
>
> (Löwith, 1997, p.52)

By giving meaning to human existence, the ascetic ideal succeeded in holding in check the threat of the most "suicidal nihilism." In the last section of the essay, Nietzsche seems to confirm this view:

> Apart from the ascetic ideal, man, the human *animal*, had no meaning so far. His existence on earth contained no goal; "why man at all?" – was a question without an answer; the *will* for man … was lacking; behind every great human destiny there sounded as a refrain a yet greater "in vain!" *This* is precisely what the ascetic ideal means: that something was *lacking*, that man was surrounded by a fearful *void* – he did not know how to justify, to account for, to affirm himself; he *suffered* from the problem of his meaning.
>
> (Nietzsche, 1989, III, §28, p.162)

The ascetic ideal protects humanity from the most suicidal form of nihilism, by providing an answer to the question of existence – the only answer so far. Nietzsche stresses this point (Nietzsche, 1989, III, §28, p.162). Therefore, it becomes clear that the ascetic ideal saves the human will from the fearful void that surrounds it; it gives the will a goal, and, in this sense, it stands against its downfall into the nothing of non-existence. Yet, the question that arises at this point is whether this prospect of the death of the will – its recession to non-existence – comprises also the will to nothingness. Can we assume that the will to nothingness and the non-being of the will are one? If this was the case, the first statement of the problem, which is repeated at the end of the last section, would make no sense, since it is the will to nothingness, which still "is and remains a *will*!" that saves the will from receding into the nothing; the nihil of the will (Nietzsche, 1989, III, §28, p.163). The answer to this question is crucial because if we accept that the will to nothingness equals the nihil of the will, then we also have to assume that Christianity succeeded to combat all forms of nihilism. The latter would be seen to resurface with the devaluation of Christian moral values in modernity. However, this is not really the case. The ascetic ideal succeeded to combat the most destructive form of nihilism, but

> that willing which has taken its direction from the ascetic ideal...this horror of the senses, of reason itself, this fear of happiness and beauty...all this means...*a will to nothingness*, an aversion to life, a rebellion against the most fundamental presuppositions of life...
>
> (Nietzsche, 1989, III, §28,m pp.162–163)

Consequently, the ascetic ideal succeeded to combat suicidal nihilism, by erecting another type of nihilism: the will that wills nothingness but remains a will. In order to see how the will which is animated by the ascetic ideal is related to the problem of life, we have to examine now more closely the relation of Christian-ascetic nihilism and modern atheistic nihilism.

In his analysis of nihilism, Deleuze sets forth a distinction that clarifies decisively the above problem: "In the word nihilism – he writes – *nihil* does not signify non-being but primarily a value of nil. Life takes on a value of nil insofar as it is denied and depreciated" (1996, p.147). According to Deleuze, this depreciation of life has to be considered as the "primary and basic sense" of nihilism: its "negative sense" – i.e., the will to negate life which occurs by ascribing to it the value of nil. The second, more colloquial sense, is that of "reactive nihilism, the one that refers to the devaluation of all these values were formerly used to depreciate life: e.g., the fiction of the supersensible world in all its forms (God, essence, the good, truth)" (Deleuze, 1996, p.147). It presupposes the previous type that depreciates life and turns it into a fiction. This is because without this first type of nihilism, the devaluation of the highest values of Christian morality and religion would not have had the effect of a generalized "in vain" addressed to existence *as such.*

> Devaluation no longer signifies life taking the value of nil, the null value, but the nullity of values, of higher values ... The nothingness of the will is no longer merely a symptom of the will to nothingness, but ultimately a negation of all will, a *tedium vitae* ... this second sense would be familiar but no less incomprehensible if we did not see how it derives from and presupposes the first. Previously life was depreciated from the height of higher values, it was denied in the name of these values. Here, on the contrary, only life remains, but it is still a depreciated life which now continues in a world without values, stripped of meaning and purpose, sliding ever further towards its nothingness ... The first sense of nihilism found its principle in the will to deny as will to power. The second sense, "the pessimism of weakness", finds its principle in the reactive life completely solitary and naked, in reactive forces reduced to themselves.
>
> (Deleuze, 1996, p.148)

In the above passage Deleuze clarifies a significant yet obscure point in Nietzsche's analysis of nihilism that often passes unnoticed: namely, the distinction between Christian nihilism, or, more generally, this type of nihilism that imbues all great religions and moralities that depreciate life and becoming in the name of "higher values," and the most familiar sense of nihilism: that which is seen to arise with the "death of God" and the devaluation of all the higher values that were advocated by Christian religion and morality. It is noteworthy that for Nietzsche this second sense of nihilism – the nihilism of modernity – derives necessarily from Christian morality itself and more specifically from the belief in the value of truth. However, in relation to the problem examined here, the most important element resides in Deleuze's observation that the will to nothingness – this will that denies all value to life and life itself – is and remains a *will to power*. It is this relation between the will that denies life and the will to power which is personified, according to Nietzsche, in the ascetic priest.

Nonetheless, in order to see how the will that denies and the will to power are united in the ascetic priest, it is necessary to examine first certain points raised by Nietzsche's inquiry into the meaning of the ascetic ideal. These two inquiries – of the meaning of the ascetic ideal and that of the role of the ascetic priest – will bring us straight into the heart of the problem of life. If the ascetic ideal has succeeded in assuming such a variety of meanings for humanity, to the extent that it coincides with meaning per se, i.e., the *only* meaning of human existence so far – the ascetic priest then held a crucial role in this process of dissemination and more radically of interpretation of the world and life itself.

The mask and the cocoon: the meaning(s) of the ascetic ideal and the role of the life-denying principle within life per se

If we follow Nietzsche's analysis closely, it becomes evident that there is no such thing as *a* meaning of the ascetic ideal. If there is meaning this is both *fluid* and *plural*. The ascetic ideal will appear to have *no meaning* whatsoever for the artist, and this holds irrespectively of whether a great artist decides to pay homage to this precise ideal that contradicts the very source of artistic creation, with its slandering of sense and sensuality (Nietzsche, 1989, III, §2–5, pp.98–103). In contrast, the ascetic ideal maintains a vital importance for philosophy.

The sections that Nietzsche devotes to the meaning(s) of the ascetic ideal for philosophy and the philosopher are maybe the most intriguing in the third essay as a whole. Using the method inaugurated in the analysis of the moral evaluations of "good" and "bad," "good" and "evil" in the first essay, and the meaning of punishment in the second essay, Nietzsche distinguishes between this part which is stable and that which is fluid in the concept of the ascetic ideal. What is stable seems to be only the *form* in the same way that in the analysis of punishment the stable aspect appeared to be *custom, the act, the drama* (Nietzsche, 1989, II, §13, pp.79–80). This distinction between form and content of the ascetic ideal is not expressly discussed in the text but it is intimated. More accurately, it is a provisional distinction: the ascetic ideal is separated from virtue and, in this sense, ceases to be considered as the primordial and inalterable *content* of virtue. Ultimately, it becomes a *form*: the *mask*, the *guise* that philosophy has to assume in order to exist. In this sense, the ascetic ideal as content is subsumed by its form: it finds its meaning in serving as a temporary disguise and cocoon for the philosopher. This conclusion is reached after a series of preliminary inquiries. The first of these inquiries concerns the use of the ascetic ideal by the individual philosopher and it is precisely at this point that its meaning is severed from virtue and reveals itself instead to be a *tool* and a *symptom* of a dominating instinct. Nietzsche insists on this point:

> The three great slogans of the ascetic ideal are familiar: poverty, humility, chastity. Now take a close look at the lives of all the great, fruitful, inventive spirits: you will always encounter all three to a certain degree. *Not*, it goes without saying, as though these constituted their "virtues" – what has this kind of man to do with virtues! – but as the most appropriate and natural conditions of their *best* existence, their *fairest* fruitfulness. It is quite possible that their dominating spirituality had first to put a check on an unrestrained and irritable pride or wanton sensuality, or that it perhaps had a hard job to maintain its will to the "desert" against a love of luxury and refinement or an excessive liberty of heart and hand. But it did it, precisely because it was the dominating instinct whose demands prevailed against those of all the other instincts – it continues to do it; if it did not do it, it would not dominate. There is thus nothing of "virtue" in this.
>
> (Nietzsche, 1989, III, §8, pp.108–109)

Thus, the ascetic ideal is here a *means* for mastery; a *tool* used by the dominant instinct of spirituality to expand its power. In this sense, the inquiry into the meaning of the ascetic ideal for philosophy is related to the general theory of meaning in Nietzsche's philosophy, which finds probably its most systematic exposition in the analysis of punishment in the second essay of the *Genealogy*. There Nietzsche elaborates on the idea that meaning is more profoundly an expression of a will to power that seeks to master a "thing" by appropriating it – by overturning, exploiting and dominating pre-existing systems of power, with their own systems of rules, relations between forces, meanings and interpretations. The imposition of a new meaning, a new interpretation is the outward expression of this mastery. For this reason, Nietzsche often uses the term *symptom* when referring to meaning. It is easy to discern the analogy here between the exposition of the problem of meaning in the analysis of punishment and that of the meaning of the ascetic ideal in philosophy. Although in the latter Nietzsche uses the term dominating instinct, it is shown later in the text in what ways the will to power comes into play in philosophy, or, more accurately, into the mask and cocoon often mistaken for philosophy itself. This is the will to truth; that is, the most persistent remnant of the ascetic ideal in the present. This is because philosophy and modern science are still driven by an unconditional will to truth – the "strictest" and "most spiritual formulation" of the ascetic ideal (Nietzsche, 1989, III, §27, p.160). Conversely, due to the persistence of the ascetic ideal in the unconditional belief to the will to truth, Nietzsche questions the very *possibility* of philosophy today (Nietzsche, 1989, III, §10, p.116). In accordance with this formulation, the possibility for philosophy opens up precisely when the "will to truth" becomes conscious of itself as a problem (C.f. Nietzsche, 1989, III, §27, p.161).

Yet, if for philosophy the ascetic ideal is just a temporary and provisional form, which obstructs and finally shutters philosophical thought when it becomes the *philosopher's pose par excellence* (Nietzsche, 1989, §10, p.116), we have to see now what it becomes in the hands of the ascetic priest. In contrast to the philosopher, for whom the ascetic ideal is a *means* to attain the necessary conditions for a higher spirituality, or a temporary cloak and cocoon, the ascetic priest "possessed in this ideal not only his faith but also his *will*, his *power*, his *interest*" (Nietzsche, 1989, §11, p.116, emphases added). In this way, in the face of the ascetic priest, the life-denying principle of the ascetic ideal becomes the very aim that the will seemed to lack. The will to nothingness embodied in the ascetic priest is his own *will to power*; not only his will, but the means through which he creates a will to power for the sick, weak and underprivileged. Before we proceed, however, to see how the ascetic priest succeeds in creating a will to power in those who seem to lack it by definition (i.e. the weak, sick and underprivileged), we must examine first the role of this life-denying principle within life itself.

> So monstruous a mode of valuation stands inscribed in the history of mankind not as an exception and curiosity, but as one of the most widespread and enduring of all phenomena. Read from a distant star, the majuscule script of our earthly existence would perhaps lead to the conclusion that the earth was the distinctively *ascetic planet*, a nook of disgruntled, arrogant, and offensive creatures filled with a profound disgust at themselves, at the earth, at all life, who inflict as much pain on themselves as they possibly can out of pleasure in inflicting pain – which is probably their only pleasure. For consider how regularly and universally the ascetic priest appears in almost every age; he belongs to no one race; he prospers everywhere; he emerges from every class of society.
>
> (Nietzsche, 1989, §11, p.117)

It can be derived from the above that the ascetic priest did not emerge with Christianity. He does not belong in any particular race or class and appears at almost in every age. This life-denying principle embodied by the ascetic priest is equally present in the Vedanta philosophy and it survives, as we saw, in atheistic modernity as "will to truth." Consequently,

> it must be a necessity of the first order that again and again promotes the growth and prosperity of this *life-inimical* species – it must indeed be in the *interest of life itself* that such a self-contradictory type does not die out.
>
> (Nietzsche, 1989, §11, p.117)

As we can see, with this last statement, the relationship between the ascetic ideal *and* life appears in the inverse order. The self-contradictory type of the ascetic priest – whose entire *mode of life* and *will* aspire to master "life itself"; that is, its "most profound, powerful, and basic conditions" (Nietzsche, 1989, III, §11, pp.117–118) – appears to serve the *interest of life itself.*

> It will be immediately obvious that such a self-contradiction as the ascetic priest appears to represent, "life *against* life" is, physiologically considered and not merely psychologically, a simple absurdity. It can only be *apparent;* it must be a kind of provisional formulation, an interpretation and psychological misunderstanding of something whose real nature could not for a long time be understood or described *as it really was* – a mere word inserted into an old *gap* in human knowledge. Let us replace it with a brief formulation of the facts of the matter: *the ascetic ideal springs from the protective instinct of a degenerating life* which tries by all means to sustain itself and fight for its existence; it indicates a partial physiological obstruction and exhaustion against which the deepest instincts of life, which have remained intact, continually struggle with new expedients and devices. The ascetic ideal is such an expedient.
>
> (Nietzsche, 1989, III, §13, p.120)

When examined from the perspective of what is known today – after the decline of Christianity as dogma – the ascetic ideal is not a force hostile to life, but something that springs "from the protective instinct of a *degenerating* life" (Nietzsche, 1989, III, §13, p.120, emphasis added). Can we conclude from this that the main function of the ascetic ideal is to serve as a cure for this degenerated form of life out of which it derives? Such view of the *interest* of life appears to contradict all other analyses of the concept of life in Nietzsche's oeuvre, including other instances where Nietzsche refers to the most distinctive characteristic of life in the *Genealogy.* In Section 27 of the third essay, Nietzsche defines the law of life as that of the *necessity* of "self-overcoming" (Nietzsche, 1989, III, §27, p.161). The same conception of life is advanced also in the *Gay Science,* where life is defined as that which is "continually shedding something that wants to die" (Nietzsche, 1974, §26, p.100). This view of life is elaborated further in *Thus Spoke Zarathustra*, where Nietzsche criticizes the metaphysical conception of life as "will to existence" and affirms once again the law of self-overcoming: "And life itself told me this secret": "Behold," it said, "I am that *which must overcome itself again and again*" (Nietzsche, 1969, p.138). The primacy of self-overcoming over the instinct of self-preservation informs Nietzsche's critique of Darwin:

> The wish to preserve oneself is the symptom of a condition of distress, of a limitation of the really fundamental instinct of life which aims at *the expansion of power* and, wishing for that, frequently risks and even sacrifices self-preservation ... in nature it is not conditions of distress that are *dominant* but overflow and squandering, even to the point of absurdity. The struggle of

> existence is only an *exception,* a temporary restriction of the will to life. The great and small struggle always revolves around superiority, around growth and expansion, around power – in accordance with the will to power which is the will of life.
>
> (Nietzsche, 1974, §349, p.292)

This passage conveys Nietzsche's fundamental proposition on the nature of life, not definable as a "will to existence" and even less as will for self-preservation, but as will to power: "the unexhausted, procreating life-will" (Nietzsche, 1969, p.137).

In relation to the above, the analysis encountered earlier (tracing the origin of the ascetic ideal in the protective instinct of a degenerating life) raises more problems than those it professes to solve. If this is the case, we would also have to accept that the "curative instinct of life" (Nietzsche, 1989, III, §16, p.128) seeks to *preserve* that which is in process of degeneration. Yet, this is not really the case. In fact, it later becomes evident that the *degenerating life* that strives to sustain itself through the actions of the ascetic priest moves in the opposite direction from the *deepest instincts* of life that have remained healthy. This internal strain and opposition between the *origin* of the ascetic ideal in the weary and degenerating form of life and the actual *curative instinct* of life becomes evident through another distinction that Nietzsche introduces: the distinction between the medication provided by the ascetic priest and the actual cure of the illness.

> It goes without saying that a "medication" of this kind, a mere affect medication, cannot possibly bring about a real cure of sickness in any physiological sense; we may not even suppose that the instinct of life contemplates or intends any sort of cure.
>
> (Nietzsche, 1989, III, §16, p.128)

The ascetic priest alleviates pain; he even provides a *meaning* to pain but does not really cure it. Yet, he succeeds in saving the will. Can we then conclude that the curative instinct of life is directed towards the salvation of the human will?

The innocent and guilty means of the ascetic priest: the direction(s) of affect and the problem of strength and weakness

In the previous section, we examined the meaning of the ascetic ideal for the ascetic priest. We approached the problem of the position of the ascetic ideal within life. This exposition appeared to arrive at a dead end. The ascetic ideal, at once life expedient of and medication directed towards the *symptoms* of the illness and not its *cause*, cannot provide any cure of the sickness itself. At the same time, life itself does not intend to cure the degenerated and the weary – if indeed it has any intentions at all. Yet the ascetic priest and the ideal that he represents succeed in curing humanity from the most destructive form of nihilism and to save the human will. It is essential to see whether this last aspect responds to the curative instinct of life which leads us to examine the means employed by the ascetic priest as a physician, shepherd, and saviour of the sick herd. In this way, we will be able to see how he succeeds in saving the human will from extinction and, thereby, seek also the real the cause of the illness.

Nietzsche draws a distinction between the "innocent" and the "guilty" means used by the ascetic priest. The first aims *aim* at alleviating pain, weariness of life and the sufferers' weariness with themselves. The soothing measures comprise the concept of redemption, mystical ecstatic experiences of unification with God, the mechanical repetitive activity of work and the ethics of work (regularity, unthinking obedience, etc.) and the prescription of the *petty pleasure* (i.e., the pleasure of giving pleasure and the feeling of superiority which is involved "in all doing good, being useful, helping and rewarding") (Nietzsche, 1989, III, §18, p.135). Nietzsche sees the latter as one of the most highly valued means of opposing depression. "By prescribing 'love of the neighbour,' the ascetic priest prescribes fundamentally an excitement of the strongest, most life-affirming drive, even if in the most cautious doses – namely of the *will to power*" (Nietzsche, 1989, III, §18, p.135).

The life-affirming drive is aroused in the weak, because the *feeling of power* – which derives in turn from the feeling of superiority over those that are in a still weaker position – is inseparable, according to Nietzsche, from this insatiable and proliferating life-will – the will to power.

Nietzsche draws this connection between the feeling of power and the will to power at various instances. In his critique of the mechanistic interpretation of the world in the *Will to Power*, he defines the will to power as an "inner quality in dynamis," i.e., force (Nietzsche, 1968, §618, p.332), or, in a more explicit formulation, "the will to power not a being, not a becoming, but a *pathos* – the most elemental fact from which a becoming and effecting must emerge" (Nietzsche, 1968, §635, p.339). In his critique of the metaphysical concept of the will (the will as something simple and absolutely known by the subject), he writes:

> The will … is above all an *affect*, and specifically the affect of command. That which is termed "freedom of the will" is essentially the affect of superiority in relation to him who must obey … A man who *wills* commands something within himself that renders obedience. But now let us notice what is strangest about the will … inasmuch as in the given circumstances we are at the same time the commanding *and* the obeying parties, and as the obeying party we know the sensations of constraint, impulsion, pressure, resistance and motion, which usually begin immediately after the act of will; inasmuch as, on the other hand, we are accustomed to disregard this duality, and to deceive ourselves about it by means of the synthetic concept "I," a whole series of erroneous conclusions, and consequently of false evaluations of the will itself, has become attached to the act of willing – to such a degree that he who wills believes sincerely that

> willing *suffices* for action ... In short, he who wills believes with a fair amount of certainty that will and action are somehow one; he ascribes the success ... to the will itself, and thereby enjoys an increase of the sensation of power which accompanies all success.
>
> (Nietzsche, 1966, §19, p.26)

In the same way that the will to power is itself complex since it always involves resisting wills, "underwills and under-souls" that eventually succumb to the victorious will that masters them, the *feeling* of power is also complex: it involves at the same time the "delight of command" *and* the "sensations of constraint, impulsion, pressure, resistance and motion," the commanding *and* the obeying party; the capacity *to affect* and the capacity of *being affected.* Now, if we follow Deleuze's pertinent observation on this matter, we can see why the capacity of being affected is even more fundamental in the will to power than the capacity to affect; and also appreciate the deeper significance of the term *pathos* used by Nietzsche in the definition of the will to power encountered above. For Deleuze, the will to power manifests itself in force as *the capacity of being affected,* precisely because "the relationship between forces in each case is determined to the extent that each force is *affected* by other, inferior or superior, forces" (Deleuze, 1996, p.62).

It is noteworthy that the capacity of being affected does not refer solely to the human will. As we have seen, the definition of will to power as pathos is introduced in Nietzsche's critique of mechanism in nature. Deleuze presents the capacity of being affected in his discussion of the problem of the manifestation of the will to power in force. As indicated in the previous passage from the *Will to Power* (Nietzsche, 1968, §635, p.339), the concepts of number, the concept of the "thing," the "subject" as well as the mechanistic conception of motion between inert particles of matter (or else, things) are "phenomenal"; that is, dependent on human perception (sight and touch), and human psychology. If we eliminate what is phenomenal and dependent on our perception, "no things remain but only dynamic quanta, in relation of tension to all other dynamic quanta: their *essence* lies in their relation to all other quanta, in their "effect" upon the same" (Nietzsche, 1968, p.635).

It transpires now clearly that affectivity – the capacity of being affected – is considered by Nietzsche as *a quality of force that derives out of the very relation of the dynamic quanta with each other.* It is in this sense that Deleuze stresses the primacy of being affected over affecting. This primary character of pathos leads to a second proposition: "the capacity for being affected is not necessarily a passivity, but an *affectivity*, a sensibility, a sensation" (Deleuze, 1996, p.62). This is because the pathos in dynamis (force), or else, the will within force, is the source out of which "both becoming *and* effecting emerge" (Nietzsche, 1968, §635, p.339). Can we conclude that this capacity of being affected, this inner pathos in force, is also a characteristic of life itself? That is, its capacity to fall ill and overcome the illness and its very cause? And, if this is the case, what would be the sense of this overcoming?

The above questions cannot be answered unless we examine more thoroughly the way in which the human will is saved from extinction through the operations of the ascetic priest, the causes and extent of the disease and the meaning of cure from the perspective of life itself.

Thus, we shall return now once again to the first point – the operations of the ascetic priest on the will of the sick, weak and weary. This minimal feeling of power, introduced by the principle of the "petty pleasure," is intensified even more through the creation of communities and congregations. In these two ways, the feeling of power of the weak is intensified. Does this intensification result in strength? Nietzsche does not pose this question directly; he offers instead a direct answer.

> With the growth of the community, a new interest grows for the individual, too, and often lifts him above the most personal element in his discontent, his aversion to *himself* ... All the sick and sickly instinctively strive after a herd organization as a means of shaking off their dull displeasure and feeling of weakness: the ascetic priest divines this instinct and furthers it; wherever there are herds, it is the instinct of weakness that has willed the herd and the prudence of the priest that has organized it. For one should not overlook the fact: the strong are as naturally inclined to *separate* as the weak are to *congregate.*
>
> (Nietzsche, 1989, III, §18, pp.135–136)

The community and congregation of the weak are driven by their very weariness and exhaustion; a weariness and decline that springs from the *aversion* that the weak feel against themselves. The question now is: does the person who is in such opposition with him/herself, really possess the capacity to obey to his/her own commanding will? Can he/she experience the essential duality of the will that we encountered earlier? The relation of mastery and obedience presupposes strife between the commanding and resisting wills, or, differently put, between conflicting aims of the will. Most importantly, this inner duality of commanding and obeying presupposes, as we shall see, an affirmative stance towards the self and the two opposed parties of the will, or, more generally, the affirmation of what stands afar and apart; of that which is other and different.

As we saw previously, the strong are determined by their tendency to separate. The *drive to separate* is connected with a type of affectivity, which is altogether different from the one which determines the predominant drive of the weak to form communities and congregations. The weak unite in order to feel an increase of their power, through the collective power of the community with which they identify. This identification with the community, its collective causes and purposes *enables* the weak to *forget* their weariness and suffering. In other words, the weak unite out of a feeling of weariness with life and with themselves. Or at least they do so when weakness is united with sickliness. In contrast, the strong tend to isolate and separate from the weak and from their own kind, out of a *pathos of distance*. Thus, in the first essay, in his critique of the utilitarian explanation of the origin of the "good," Nietzsche writes:

> [T]he judgment "good" did *not* originate with those to whom "goodness" was shown! Rather it was "the good" themselves, that is to say, the noble, powerful, high-stationed and high-minded, who felt and established themselves and their actions as good, that is, of the first rank, in contradiction to all the low, low-minded, common and plebeian. In was out of this *pathos of distance* that they first seized the right to create values and to coin names for values: what had they to do with utility! The viewpoint of utility is as remote and inappropriate as it possibly could be in face of such burning eruption of the highest rank-ordering, rank-defining value judgments: for here feeling has attained the antithesis of that low degree of warmth which any calculating prudence, any calculus of utility, presupposes.
>
> (Nietzsche, 1989, I, §2, pp.25–26)

Even before they create values and names for values, the strong, noble and powerful are distinguished precisely through their pathos – the pathos of distance – which is both creative *and* affirmative: it creates distance and even difference, through an affirmative act. Moreover, the creation of values here at stake emerges out of a high feeling – high in tension and power of eruption – as against plebeian thought and its calculating prudence. It is in this higher type of affectivity that the term "strong" finds its full meaning. In support of this view in Chapter 9, Section 257 of *Beyond Good and Evil,* we read:

> Without the *pathos of distance* which grows out of the ingrained difference between strata – when the ruling caste looks afar and looks down upon subjects and instruments and just as constantly practices obedience and command, keeping down and keeping at a distance – that other, more mysterious pathos could not have grown up either – the craving for an ever new widening of distances within the soul itself, the development of ever higher, rarer, more remote, further-stretching, more comprehensive states – in brief, simply the enhancement of the type "man," the continual "self-overcoming of man," to use a moral formula in a supra-moral sense. To be sure, one should not yield to humanitarian illusions about the origins of an aristocratic society … In the beginning, the noble caste was always the barbarian caste: their predominance did not lie mainly in physical strength but in strength of the soul – they were more *whole* human beings (which also means, at every level, "more whole beasts").
>
> (Nietzsche, 1966, §257, pp.201–202)

In the last phrase of the above passage, it is clearly indicated that strength is a matter of the soul – of the ever higher, rarer, more remote and more comprehensive states – despite the fact that in the first part, it is clearly stated that this "widening of distances within the soul itself" could not take place without this primary and "external" manifestation of distance between the ruling, noble castes and the "subjects" and "instruments." The order between the first and the second form of distance cannot be overlooked. For if the distance between the strong and the weak, the noble and the vulgar, assumes an external form in the first essay of the *Genealogy*, in the second essay, it becomes the condition for the emergence of "the gravest and uncanniest illness, from which humanity has not yet recovered, man's suffering *of man, of himself...*" (Nietzsche, 1989, II, §16, p.85). Yet this point cannot be apprehended in its full sense if we do not examine first the relationship between the strong and the weak from the perspective of weakness.

The weak, or more accurately, the priestly mode of valuation, springs also from an affect and in fact, one of the strongest and most dangerous affects; that is, *ressentiment*

> The slave revolt in morality begins when *ressentiment* itself becomes creative and gives birth to values: the *ressentiment* of natures that are denied the true reaction, that of deeds, and compensate themselves with an imaginary revenge. While every noble morality develops from a triumphant affirmation of itself, slave morality from the outset says No to what is "outside," what is "different," what is "not itself"; and *this* No is its creative deed. This inversion of the value-positing eye – this need to direct one's view outward instead of back to oneself – is of the essence of *ressentiment*: in order to exist, slave morality always first needs a hostile external world; it needs, psychologically speaking, external stimuli in order to act at all – its action is fundamentally reaction.
>
> (Nietzsche, 1989, I, §10, pp.36–37)

The priestly mode of valuation, which is the motive force of the slave revolt in morality, derives from a totally different type of affectivity and an inverse perspective from the noble system of evaluation. The two – the noble valuation with its pathos of distance and the slave morality driven by ressentiment – remain inverse all the way through precisely because they originate from and move in an altogether different type of affectivity. For this reason, the mode of valuation of the weak might be victorious, but this victory does not alter at all the fact of weakness. Inversely, although *ressentiment* is the type of affectivity which is distinctive of the weak, it is one of the most dangerous and destructive weapons. It is precisely this weapon which is used by the ascetic priest in the third essay as the most effective expedient for opposing the feeling of weariness with life and with themselves of those who are sick.

> To wrench the human soul from its moorings, to immerse it in terrors, ice, flames and ruptures to such an extent that it is liberated from all petty displeasure, gloom, depression as by a flash of lightning...Fundamentally, every great affect has this power, provided it explodes suddenly...and the ascetic priest has indeed pressed into his service indiscriminately the *whole* pack of savage hounds in man and let loose now this one and now that, always with the same end in view: to awaken men from their slow melancholy, to hunt away, if only for a time, their dull pain and lingering misery...
>
> (Nietzsche, 1989, III, §20, pp.139–140)

In other words, in order to save the human will from extinction, the ascetic priest has produced "orgies of feeling" in the souls of the sick. Certainly, such orgy of feeling did not cure the sick: it rather attenuated the illness (Nietzsche, 1989, III, §20, p.140). Yet, at the same time, he *through this operation, the ascetic priest*, rendered the sick and illness itself harmless for life. This is because the ascetic priest *changed the direction of ressentiment*. Instead of being turned towards everyone which stands outside, to those who are different and stand apart from the community of the weak, ressentiment was finally directed against the sufferers themselves.

> Man, suffering from himself...like an animal shut up in a cage, uncertain why or wherefore, thirsting for reasons...thirsting, too, for remedies and narcotics, at last he takes counsel with one who knows hidden things, too – and behold! He receives a hint, he receives from his sorcerer, the ascetic priest, the *first* hint as to the "cause" of his suffering: he must seek it in *himself*, in some *guilt*, in a piece of the past, he must understand his suffering as a *punishment*. He has heard, he has understood, this unfortunate: from now on he is like a hen imprisoned by a chalk line. He can no longer get out of this chalk circle: the invalid has been transformed into "the sinner."
>
> (Nietzsche, 1989, III, §20, pp.140–141)

This change in the direction of ressentiment, which finally gave a *meaning* to suffering, occurs with the Christian version of the ascetic ideal. Hence also its tremendous importance: by redirecting the movement of ressentiment to the sufferers themselves, it safeguarded the ascending, healthy and strong instincts of life from being contaminated. Moreover, it saved the human will from extinction. Yet, it did not eradicate the cause of the illness.

Nietzsche gives various hints as to where we *should not* look for the causes of the illness. As he shows, "guilt," "sin," "punishment" are misinterpretations of the real causes and nature of suffering. Yet, he also points the direction where the real causes, as well as the origin of the illness, might be seen to reside. As he writes, "the chief trick of the ascetic priest" was "the exploitation of the *sense of guilt*" (Nietzsche, 1989, III, §20, p.140), intimating by this the sense of guilt *before* it was turned into sin. This point is extensively examined in the second essay of the *Genealogy*. As Nietzsche shows, the concept of guilt originates in the juridical system of the first contractual relations between the creditor and the debtor. However, the *sense of guilt*, that is, guilt internalized, occurs with the emergence of bad conscience. It is there in this latter line of descent, that we encounter the cause of the "gravest and uncanniest illness, from which humanity has not yet recovered, man's suffering *of man, of himself*" (Nietzsche, 1989, II, §16, p.85). The origins and causes of this illness that inflicts *humanity* as such lie in the enclosure of humankind within the walls of society and civilization. But this was not merely a physical enclosure: the taming of the "animal man" occurred first, by changing the direction of instincts; instead of being turned outwards into actions and deeds, they were turned against themselves. The origin of bad conscience lies in this hindering and redirection of the instincts against the person who has them. The cause of this illness lies neither in the ascetic priest, or the priestly mode of valuation that we encountered previously in our discussion of the distinction between the strong and the weak, the noble and plebeian. It is rather the strong themselves, the artists with the "look of bronze" that restricted and made latent the "instinct for freedom," or, more to the point, the will to power, and turned its direction inwards. In this way, the strong, noble and high-minded artists created, out of their pathos for distance, also the conditions for this other more mysterious pathos, "the craving for an ever-new widening of distances within the soul itself" (Nietzsche, 1966, §257, p.201). This double perspective of the "internalization of man" (Nietzsche, 1998, II, §16, p.84) manifests the common origin of sickness – the fearful void that surrounds human existence and the problem of the meaning of suffering – and the self-overcoming of man. It is in this second sense that this

> uncanny, dreadful joyous labor of a soul at odds with itself … eventually this entire *active* "bad conscience" – you will have guessed it – as the womb of all ideal and imaginative phenomena, also brought to light an abundance of strange new beauty and affirmation, and perhaps beauty itself.
>
> (Nietzsche, 1989, II, §18, pp.87–88)

References

Deleuze, G. (1996). *Nietzsche and Philosophy*. (H. Tomlinson, trans.) London: The Anthlone Press.

Foucault, M. (1996). *Nietzsche, Genealogy, History* in *Language, Counter-Memory, Practice: Selected Essays and Interviews*. (D.F.Bouchard, ed. D. F. Bouchard & S. Simon trans.) Ithaca, NY: Cornell University Press.

Löwith, K. (1997). *Nietzsche's Philosophy of the Eternal Recurrence of the Same*. (J. Harvey Lomax, trans.) Berkeley, Los Angeles, London: University of California Press.

Nietzsche, F. (1974). *The Gay Science*. (W. Kaufmann, trans.) New York: Vintage Books.

Nietzsche, F. (1966). *Beyond Good and Evil*. (W. Kaufmann, trans.) New York: Vintage Books.

Nietzsche, F. (1968). *The Will to Power*. (W. Kaufmann, R. J. Hollingdale, trans.) New York: Vintage Books.

Nietzsche, F. (1969). *Thus Spoke Zarathustra*. (R. J. Hollingdale, trans.) London: Penguin Books.

Nietzsche, F. (1989). *On the Genealogy of Morals*. (W. Kauffman, trans.) NewYork: Vintage Books.

Reginster, B. (2021). *The Will to Nothingness: An Essay on Nietzsche's On the Genealogy of Morality*. Oxford: Oxford University Press.

Scheler, M. (1975). *Ressentiment*. (L. Coser, ed. W. Holdheim, trans.) New York: Schocken Books.

Chapter 10

Therapy, outside

Emily Corrie

When I was a trainee therapist, I walked each week to my personal therapy sessions. The route took about 47 minutes, and much of it passed through London's beautiful Hampstead Heath and Highgate Wood to the north. I had always loved to walk, and I enjoyed this opportunity before my sessions to reconnect and reconsider myself among the swaying grasses and old trees. One day, in my first semester of training, I slumped onto my therapist's couch and lamented the fact that I would have to sit for the next 50 minutes and talk. I was tired of talking. The existential philosophers I had come to London to study—Nietzsche, Kierkegaard, Sartre—sang an anthem of action and courage. "We do not belong to those who have ideas only among books," counselled Nietzsche:

> It is our habit to think outdoors—walking, leaping, climbing, dancing, preferably on lonely mountains or near the sea where even the trails become thoughtful. Our first questions about the value of a book, of a human being, or a musical composition are: Can they walk? Even more, can they dance?
>
> (Gros, 2014, p. 18)

But studying existential psychotherapy, I had disappointedly discovered, involved sitting, talking, and reading rather than leaping, climbing, and dancing. My therapist, after listening to my complaints, cast a glance outside and said: "Okay, let's go for a walk". Yet despite my boredom at the thought of sitting politely for another hour talking, and despite my restless desire to challenge and question traditional ways of doing therapy, I was suddenly afraid of the prospect of going out into the "real world" with my therapist. Who would we each be out there? What might happen? I did not find out. I stayed sitting on that couch and talked for the necessary 50 minutes: I played the therapy game. I wish I had gotten off that couch and embraced the uncertainty. I was, and still am, embarrassed that I had not had the courage to try something different.

What I had been restlessly craving was a more natural—human?—way of doing and experiencing therapy. Indeed, it was always the humanness of the interaction—the strange intimacy, the immediacy—that intrigued me about the enterprise and provoked me to embark on psychotherapy training in the first place.

DOI: 10.4324/9781003669906-11

Two people, confronted with one another. Two people talking, sure, but how often did the talking become an excuse? A distraction from what was actually physically happening: two bodies meeting in space. Bruno Latour (2004) suggests

> to have a body is to learn to be affected, meaning 'effectuated', moved, put into motion by other entities, humans or nonhumans. If you are not engaged in this learning, you become insensitive, dumb, you drop dead.
>
> (p. 205)

In psychotherapy, "affect" tends to be conflated with emotion—and usually always the client's emotion. The aim of Affect Therapy, for example, is to help clients access and experience their blocked emotions. But to be a therapist or a client is also an affective experience—we are, inevitably, affected by one another. It seems strange that we can focus so much on the content matter of the sessions—the client's verbal or emotional expressions—but ignore (or, indeed, avoid) the very fact of the encounter itself.

Years after being too afraid to get off my therapist's couch and go outside, I found myself living on a large farm in a leafy, relatively empty part of France. It offered the perfect setting for outdoor therapy. My first experiences as a newly accredited therapist working outside with clients became the basis for my dissertation: an autoethnographic exploration of walk-and-talk therapy. What I discovered when I took therapy outside went some way to answering my questioning over why I tended to allow myself to be distracted by the verbal and emotional content of therapy sessions: because the encounter is unsettling. To be affected is scary.

During the first two months that I offered walk-and-talk therapy, I kept weekly journal entries about my experience bringing therapy outside. My first reflections were preoccupied with how different therapy looked outside. Normally, therapy sessions are conducted in a contained and intimate setting. For example, Knox and Cooper (2015) advise that "therapy rooms should be a calm, clear and clean environment. … Seating should be comfortable, with no harsh lighting (but not romantically dark either!), and the room should also be at a comfortable temperature" (p. 2). Such a setting is intended to make the client feel safe: here in this secure room, away from prying eyes and the distractions of the world outside, she can reveal her secrets. But the room also makes the *therapist* feel safe. The room is the therapist's room, after all, into which the client enters. The therapist is in control of the seating arrangement, the temperature, the lighting, and the decor. The therapist has carefully arranged clocks so that the time might be easily tracked by both therapist and client, and the finiteness of their relationship is therefore clearly on display. The therapist's choice of rugs and paintings reflects her beliefs about how much of her personal life and style she will reveal to her client. In her therapy room (or Zoom room), the therapist can be secure, undistracted by her life (and self) outside the walls; here she can play the role of "therapist". Taking therapy outside means that the therapist meets the client on equal ground. Although the therapist will have already mapped out a route, the walking trails do not belong to her, and the natural world cannot be manipulated and controlled for her therapeutic purposes. The natural world exists separate from the purpose of the therapy session. The therapist and client must strike out together, both uncertain of what they will find.

The move outside can shift usual assumptions of hierarchy and authority. Different therapists navigate this in different ways. Some therapists choose to fashion outdoor therapy spaces that mirror indoor spaces, such as Jordan (2013) who constructed a dome made from willow branches. The room itself was made of natural material and in an outdoor setting, but it was protected from the weather and seasons and provided a sense of confidentiality, privacy, and control over the environment. For some therapists, see an outdoor therapy space fashioned like this as only a half-move outside. The point of doing therapy outside is that it offers a chance to "shake up" the traditional roles of therapist and client.

I am not the first therapist to have documented the uncertainty that arises when working outside the therapy room. The absence of an established theoretical base, limited access to specialist supervision, and a lack of formal training institutions are difficulties that outdoor therapists frequently point to (Revell & McLeod, 2017; McKinney, 2011). As one therapist stated, "For a lot of things, I just make it up as I go" (McKinney, 2011, p. 98). For me, this move outside was disconcerting, and I was hyper aware of certain elements of "frame" that, outside, became loose and untamable and that made me feel uncomfortably out of control. The weather, for example, made me question what I was supposed to wear as a walk-and-talk therapist. Was it okay to wear shorts when the sun was blazing? When we are in a group, we tend to adapt our clothing to those around us—either by adopting the same general styles, or countering them. But as a walk-and-talk therapist, I was alone and uncertain of what was considered "normal". I wanted a uniform and the comfort that wearing it would give me.

Time was another element of frame that brought vulnerability. Unlike when we are sitting in a traditional therapy room, where it is possible to track the clock and usher the client out of the room or click the "end call" button perfectly on time, when we are outside and moving, the end of a session is marked by completing the walking loop. Indeed, midway through the session we might be many kilometres away from the client's car. The length of a session is therefore measured not only by the minute hand on the clock but also by distance, pace, and weather. During one walk-and-talk therapy session, I realized that I had forgotten to bring a phone or watch to track the time. Initially, I panicked and felt out of control. I wondered what my client would think of my competencies as a therapist if we arrived back at his car either much too early or much too late. Of course, I had no option but to continue the route that we had begun. When we arrived back, I discovered that the session had, in the end, been timed perfectly. Since then, I no longer rigidly adhere to clock time but instead time sessions by the route and the pace at which we walk.

Perhaps the most glaring difference I found in beginning to work outside was the amount of myself that was on display to my clients. When I am outside walking next to them, my clients are privy to aspects of my self-as-human that my non-walking clients are not. They know, for example, my walking speed and style, how I respond to weather, and how I interact with unexpected events that happen along the way. I am a human who moves around in the world, not just a face on a screen or a therapist sitting in a chair. My choice to start and end my walking therapy sessions from my farm also means that lines sometimes blur between my self-as-therapist and self-as-farmer. My farming life inserts itself into sessions whether I choose for it to or not; the trail we walk along borders one of my fields where my cows, sheep, and horses graze, and sometimes one of my dogs invites itself along for sessions. Initially, this blurring of worlds made me feel uncomfortable, and I did not know how to navigate it. I remember one session when my client arrived early and was waiting on the bench outside my home. When I came out to join him, I noticed that my goats had escaped and were spread out everywhere on the road in front of my house, wreaking havoc on the grapes and flowers. My journal entry from that day's session described the incident:

> Now I'm a farmer in front of my client, herding up goats and asking my dog to drive them into their pen. My client helps by dragging one goat by its horns. A strange therapy, this. Some part of me is questioning if this is normal or if I am committing some great therapy crime. But another larger part accepts that this is the therapy that I offer: Sometimes we talk; sometimes we herd goats.
>
> (Personal journal, 20 October 2022)

At another point, I remember walking with a client past the late-summer vegetable garden and feeling incredibly embarrassed that my tomato plants had all fallen from their stakes in a wild mess. Knowing that the client was also a gardener, I wondered if they would question the therapeutic capacities of someone who gardened so messily. Yet despite my initial uneasiness of allowing these messy farmer realities to be on display, I have also found that my walking therapy clients (who are themselves often farmers) cite the fact that I am a farmer as the reason why they chose me as their therapist, and that it puts them at ease to be outside in the open air in a familiar setting. Indeed, often the messiness and unpredictability of a farming life becomes part of the therapeutic conversation itself.

The growing field of ecopsychology considers that a recognition of the interconnectivity of nature is essential to human well-being. Ecopsychotherapists tend to therefore "use" nature in the sessions, such as by making connections between the client's words and the natural world or by more active exercises such as using objects found in nature (sticks, rocks, leaves), as a way to help clients express their inner experience (Berger, 2008). Ecopsychotherapists therefore use nature as a tool or partner in the therapy. In my search for some certainty and some sense that I was "doing it right", I felt like I was somehow failing as a walk-and-talk therapist if the natural world wasn't more explicitly present in the conversation. The efforts I had made to do this felt forced and *unnatural*. Near the end of one session, during which I had been quietly feeling awkward about this perceived lack in my therapeutic capacities, my client told me that before the session he had felt anxious about what to talk about in the session and how he could "make the most of it". But, he explained, when he had started to walk, the words had come out and the conversation had happened without effort. His words were learning for me, too. Both of us had been feeling anxious about how we might be able to control the session and "use" it for a certain aim. But once our feet started to move, the session unfolded as it did; as it always does. We each only had to trust that something would happen, one step at a time.

Gradually, working outside taught me to begin to let go of my control and to trust in the process. Although of course even when we are seated in our therapy rooms or in front of a computer screen, things arise from the outside (or inside) world that we must navigate, I have found that these occurrences are more obviously on display when working outside, where our environment is not managed for our therapeutic purposes and exists in its own accord. I found that these occurrences are opportunities to decide how I want to act—both as a therapist and as a human. In one memorable session, I had the urge to stop to pick a particularly juicy-looking blackberry. My urge made me pause and contemplate whether it would be appropriate to respond to it—I would not get up in the middle of a therapy session to peel open a tablet of chocolate, after all. In that moment of decision, standing in front of the blackberry bushes, I had a memory of going to a meditation group, once, and, after having sat motionless facing an electrical socket on the wall for the previous hour, I had had the urge to burst out laughing. I had not laughed, however, because I did not think it was permitted, and I had continued to sit stoically in silence. I had always wondered what would have happened if I had allowed myself to laugh. Thinking about that memory, I reached for the blackberry. No one had ever instructed me: "Thou shalt not pick blackberries with clients", and yet I felt somehow penned in by unspoken rules. My decision to pick the blackberry was a decision to act and see what would happen. It was also an expression of my desire to question the usual conventions we operate within.

As an existentially trained therapist, I am no stranger to the idea of uncertainty. Indeed, it was a desire to confront and steep myself in uncertainty that inspired me to train as a therapist in the first place. For Spinelli (2015), uncertainty is one of the defining principles of existential psychotherapy. "The principle of uncertainty," Spinelli writes, "asserts that I can never fully determine with complete and final certainty or control not only what will present itself as stimulus to my experience, but also how I will experience and respond to stimuli" (2015, p. 22). The fact that I live in a world populated by the rest of nature (humans, animals, plants) means that I am always in relation to other beings, navigating and responding to them. As a therapist, I am confronted with the uncertainty of being in relation to another human. This uncertainty begins when a new client contacts me for a first session. I can never know whom I will meet on that first day, or what they will want to tell me. Of course, this is also the case for clients I have already met many times before, but my assumptions and preconceptions have a habit of leaping in to limit the sense of uncertainty I feel. To honour another human is to give up my control and allow myself to be continuously surprised by the encounter. Such surprise is disconcerting and uncomfortable. I might try to control this discomfort by ascribing to a certain therapeutic method as a sort of guidebook to orient me, adopting techniques to aid my behaviour, and developing a set of habits that make me feel safe. In a therapy context, these efforts serve to make me feel—and present myself—like I am a capable professional. Without them, I might feel useless and powerless, and, worse yet, my client might have the same suspicions of me. Spinelli (2001) likens these sorts of customs to "magic feathers"—in reference to Disney's Dumbo who believed he was only able to fly because he possessed a magic feather—and urges practitioners to take note of what magic feathers are holding up their therapy practice. As therapists, we ask our clients every day to brave the uncertainty that accompanies taking a hard look at their usual habits and assumptions, and the unsettledness of their finite life. Yet as therapists we are often rigidly confined to our habits and assumptions of what therapy is and what it should look like (and where it should be conducted). Stepping outside the therapy room and exploring how I exist in relation to my client while working outside in nature made me more aware of the magic feathers that I possess.

The uncertainty I felt while working outside was of the existential variety, too. Lacking the familiar confines of a therapy room and the frame it provides, I found myself questioning the very enterprise of therapy: what is it for? What is my role as a therapist? I felt unsettled without having clear and established answers to these questions. Schneider (2015) notes that arguably most of our troubles as humans "are traceable to one overriding problem: our suspension in the groundlessness of existence" (p. 21). In *The Wisdom of Insecurity*, Watts (1951/2011) argues that it is contradictory to desire security in a universe that is fluid and changing. A desire to seek safety and avoid the flux of life is also a desire to be separate from life. But it is in this separateness that we feel insecure: "To be secure means to isolate and fortify the 'I', but it is just the feeling of being an isolated 'I' which makes me feel lonely and afraid" (Watts, 1951/2022, p. 77). When I stepped outside the traditional therapy room, I felt distractingly aware of my uncertainty in this new environment. Yet I discovered that despite my desire to control the therapy sessions—particularly by explicitly drawing attention to the natural world through which we walked—it was when I relinquished control and allowed the session to flow of its own accord that I felt most present and the least uncertain. When I felt most present, I also felt least alone; I became aware of my interconnection with the client by my side and the living world through which we walked.

In his *A Philosophy of Walking*, Fredric Gros (2014) makes the obvious claim that everyone knows how to walk

> You don't learn how to walk … there is no technique, no panic about getting it right or not, about doing it this way rather than that, no pressure to pull yourself together, practice, concentrate. Everyone knows how to walk. One foot in front of the other.
>
> (p. 35)

For these reasons, walking, I would argue, presents a beautiful metaphor for our work as therapists. For me, doing therapy outside has been a lesson in giving up control and a reminder that therapy, like life, is a journey without a particular destination. These were ideas that inspired me to become a therapist in the first place: a desire to embrace uncertainty and make it the practice of my life and profession. But of course uncertainty is scary, and it's easy to become distracted by the idea that a certain technique, or tool, or method can be the answer (an answer for our client's suffering, but also our own suffering as their uncertain therapist). Working outside was a literal stepping outside my usual ways of working and the usual therapeutic frame: a step into the unknown. The rules that guided me seemed suddenly flimsy and out of context; instead, I was presented with a real, living, breathing, changing world which inspired me—and forced me—to be myself: a real, living, breathing human in an encounter with another.

References

Berger, R. (2008). Building a home in nature: An innovative framework for practice. *Journal of Humanistic Psychology, 48*(2), pp. 264–279.

Gros, F. (2014). *A philosophy of walking.* London and New York: Verso.

Jordan, M. (2013). *Taking therapy outside: A narrative inquiry into counselling and psychotherapy in outdoor natural spaces.* [Unpublished doctoral dissertation]. University of Brighton.

Knox, R., and Cooper, M. (2015). *The therapeutic relationship in counselling and psychotherapy.* London: Sage.

Latour, B. (2004). How to talk about the body? The normative dimension of science studies. *Body & Society, 10*(2–3), pp. 205–229.

Mckinney, B.L. (2011). *Therapist's perceptions of walk and talk therapy: A grounded study.* [Unpublished doctoral dissertation]. University of New Orleans.

Revell, S., and McLeod, J. (2017). Therapists' experience of walk and talk therapy: A descriptive phenomenological study. *European Journal of Psychotherapy and Counselling, 19*(3), pp. 267–289.

Schneider, K.J. (2015). The case for existential (spiritual) psychotherapy. Journal of Contemporary Psychotherapy, 45, pp. 21–24.

Spinelli, E. (2001). *The mirror and the hammer.* London: Continuum.

Spinelli, E. (2015). *Practicing existential therapy,* 2nd edition. London: Sage

Watts, A. (1951/2011). *The wisdom of insecurity: A message for an age of anxiety.* New York: Vintage.

Chapter 11

Life, truth, and exception in Badiou's *Logics of Worlds*

Michalis Tegos

Introduction

In *Logics of Worlds*, Alain Badiou foregrounds a distinctive and provocative account of exceptionality that spans the full arc of the book. Central to this philosophical trajectory is the unexpected role played by the concept of "life." While often framed as the paradigm of continuity, regularity, and universality—a category that admits no exception—life, for Badiou, becomes the very site where a *logic of exception* can be most radically staged. This move is anything but accidental. As Badiou is well aware, "life" is not a neutral term within the landscape of contemporary philosophy. It serves, rather, as a privileged concept in a broader philosophical lineage that includes Nietzsche, Bergson, and Deleuze—a vitalist tradition that Badiou identifies as deeply anti-Platonic. Against this dominant current of 20th-century French thought, which posits life in terms of affect, embodiment and wellbeing, Badiou positions his own project as an explicit intervention: one that seeks to reaffirm the Platonic legacy of philosophy by reasserting the primacy of truth, fidelity, and exception over the flux of becoming and the immanence of life.

Badiou's Platonism and the tradition of vitalism

At the heart of Badiou's polemic is a simple but profound claim: that philosophy, if it is to remain philosophy, must remain tethered to the category of *truth*. Philosophy does not itself produce truths; rather, it acts as a reflective and systematizing discourse that draws its vitality from truths produced in extra-philosophical domains—namely, science, art, politics, and love. This structural dependence of philosophy on these four conditions constitutes the core of Badiou's philosophical formalism (Badiou, 1989).

This commitment to truth, however, places Badiou in direct opposition to what he sees as the dominant ideological configuration of the contemporary world: what he calls *democratic materialism*. The axiom of democratic materialism is, according to Badiou (2009, p. 4), deceptively simple: "There are only bodies and languages." This materialist slogan privileges lived experience, embodiment,

DOI: 10.4324/9781003669906-12

and discursive plurality over any commitment to universal truth. And it is this reduction—of thought to language, of being to bodies, and of ethics to life—that Badiou seeks to contest.

Democratic materialism, in his view, does not merely reject Platonism; it rejects, as we shall see below, the very structure of exception and fidelity that truth presupposes. As such, it constitutes not merely an anti-Platonic stance, but an anti-philosophical one. To live "without ideas," which is the maxim of democratic materialism, Badiou argues, is not merely to abandon a particular philosophical school—it is to abandon philosophy itself.

This tension culminates in what might be seen as a kind of philosophical scandal: the decision to conclude *Logics of Worlds* with the question, "What is it to live?" For a philosopher so rigorously aligned with abstraction, formalization, and mathematical ontology, this return to the category of life is both surprising and significant.

Indeed, Badiou himself acknowledges the apparent contradiction. Life, after all, has long been handed over to the camp of his adversaries—the vitalists, the phenomenologists, culturalists and relativists, the philosophers of affect and embodiment. Within the logic of democratic materialism, life is the highest value, the ground of all meaning and ethics. And yet, Badiou reclaims life—not by subsuming it within his ontology, but by reframing it within a *logic of exception*.

This is where Badiou's concept of the *materialist dialectic* becomes crucial. While the term recalls the tradition of dialectical materialism associated with Marxism and with Badiou's own teacher, Louis Althusser, Badiou's version is distinctive (2012b). His materialist dialectic begins not from the continuity of historical processes or the dialectical movement of material forces, but from the rupture introduced by an event. It is a dialectic of discontinuity, fidelity, and subtraction—a logic in which the exception, rather than the rule, becomes the motor of transformation.

Badiou's engagement with life is not a return to vitalism, but a polemical repurposing of its terms. Life is not the flux of becoming, but the site in which an exception may take place. It is not the horizon of immanence, but the space of its interruption.

Badiou's treatment of life in *Logics of Worlds* thus demands a re-evaluation of its place within philosophical discourse. Far from being a marginal or external concern, life is revealed as a key battleground in the struggle over the future of philosophy itself. For Badiou, the true question is not how to affirm life, but how to interrupt it: how to identify and remain faithful to those exceptional events that break with the continuity of lived experience and orient it toward truth. In this sense, life is not what philosophy affirms, but what it must subtract from—in order to think. And it is precisely in this subtraction, this logic of exception, that Badiou reasserts the vocation of philosophy as the discipline of truths.

To grasp the full philosophical significance of Badiou's intervention, we must revisit the ancient distinction between *zoē* and *bios*—biological life versus the good life. While *zoē* designates life in its most generic, animal sense—life as mere survival—*bios* refers to a qualified form of life, a life of flourishing (*eudaimonia*), guided by ethical commitments and the pleasures of philosophical thought, a life worth living. Ancient philosophy, from Aristotle to the Stoics, variously explored this distinction. Though Badiou rarely draws directly from Aristotle or Stoic ethics, his invocation of life in *Logics of Worlds* implicitly revives this classical problem, if in a highly unorthodox form.

In our contemporary predicament, however, the line between *zoē* and *bios* has all but collapsed. The good life has been displaced by the imperative to survive. Philosophical reflection on *how* one ought to live has been supplanted by concern *that* one continues to live—a condition Badiou diagnoses as symptomatic of democratic materialism. His challenge is not merely to revive the question of the good life but to radicalize it: to show that life, in the philosophical sense, becomes meaningful only when interrupted by an event that introduces the possibility of an eternal truth.

Indeed, one of the defining claims of Badiou's mature philosophy is that truths are eternal, even if their emergence is contingent (Badiou, 2009, p. 513). A truth does not derive from life, nor from biological continuity, but instead breaks into a situation from *outside* its governing logic. This is what Badiou names an *event*—an incalculable rupture that reconfigures the coordinates of the possible. It is only in fidelity to such an event that a subject is formed and that life is reorganized in light of something other than its own repetition.

This is also why Badiou sees contemporary vitalism—especially in its Deleuzian, Bergsonian, or Nietzschean guises—not merely as philosophically misguided, but as metaphysically *conformist*. The vitalist affirmation of becoming, immanence, and life as creative force ultimately remains enclosed within the logic of the world it seeks to affirm. For Badiou, it is precisely the *exception* to life, the cut in its continuity, that makes philosophical subjectivity possible. As he provocatively asserts, "humanity" is not a natural species, but rather a category retroactively produced through fidelity to truths (Badiou, 2009, 2007).

Badiou's concept of *democratic materialism* crystallizes this concern. According to its central axiom—"there are only bodies and languages"—nothing transcends the material and discursive composition of a given world. All positions are equally valid, all expressions reducible to particularity, all bodies interchangeable. Democratic materialism thus appears tolerant, open, and egalitarian. But for Badiou, this vision masks a deep nihilism: a denial of the very dimension that permits rupture, transcendence, and subjective transformation.

The "democratic" aspect of this materialism refers to the horizontal equivalence of opinions—the leveling of all thought to perspective, all truth to discourse. "Materialism" names the reduction of being to embodied existence—bodies as loci of sensation, affect, and survival. What is excluded from this vision is precisely what Badiou takes to be most essential: the ability of the subject to *exceed* its material determination by affirming the consequences of a truth that is not reducible to its body or its language.

This is where Badiou's Platonism finds its critical edge, as he finds in Plato the resources to think the human as *that which can participate in eternity*. Yet, the eternal is not elsewhere, but immanent in the event that interrupts the ordinary. In fidelity to this event, the subject becomes something more than a living being—it becomes a finite fragment of an infinite truth.

This Platonism is then neither a metaphysical mysticism nor an ethical puritanism. Rather, it is a political and ontological wager: that human beings are capable of breaking from the inertia of their world, and that philosophy's task is to think the consequences of such breaks. It is here that Badiou's divergence from Deleuze becomes most pointed. Deleuze's anti-Platonism valorizes immanence, becoming, and the creativity of life itself. For Badiou, however, such a position fails to account for the moment of rupture that distinguishes truth from novelty, fidelity from spontaneity, and subjectivation from mere transformation.

In *Deleuze: The Clamor of Being*, Badiou makes a remark—half serious, half ironic—that what held Deleuze back, in Badiou's eyes, was his anti-Platonism, his refusal to affirm the Platonic schema of eternal truth. In Deleuze's relentless celebration of difference, becoming, and immanence, Badiou sees a missed opportunity: the failure to formulate a theory of the event capable of grounding a universal and subtractive truth.

To understand why this failure matters, we must recall that for Badiou, philosophy exists only insofar as it organizes the consequences of such truths. It does not create them, nor does it merely describe the world. Rather, it reflects upon the implications of those rare moments when the world is changed by the emergence of something wholly new—a new theory in science, a new form in art, a new procedure in politics, a new fidelity in love. These are not mere intensifications of life, but *exceptions* to it.

Badiou's Platonism, then, is not antiquated but strategic. It seeks to recover a philosophical orientation that is capable of resisting the reductions imposed by democratic materialism and vitalist immanence alike. His wager is that only a philosophy grounded in the event, and organized through the categories of truth and subjectivity, can reclaim the possibility of the good life—not as pleasure or flourishing, but as fidelity to what exceeds the human and reconfigures its possibilities.

The event in Deleuze

A pivotal axis of Badiou's project in *Logics of Worlds* is his sustained engagement with Gilles Deleuze—an engagement that is at once philosophical confrontation and conceptual expropriation. As the reader moves into the second half of *Logics of Worlds*, it becomes increasingly clear that Badiou is staging his own system in deliberate opposition to Deleuze's metaphysics.

The central issue in this confrontation concerns the category of the *event*. Badiou identifies what he sees as a fundamental equivocation in Deleuze's thought: the conflation of being, life, and event under a single ontological figure—what Deleuze sometimes names as the *One*. According to Badiou, Deleuze ultimately sketches a vision in which all difference, all becoming, all intensive variation are already internal to being—a being that is not substance or identity, but pure multiplicity, pure flux. In this model, the event does not interrupt being; it is *immanent* to being.

The event is not a rupture but a modulation of life's intensive processes. In short: for Deleuze, there is no ontological distance between life, being, and the event. This, for Badiou, is precisely the problem.

Badiou's own conceptual edifice is centered on the disjunction of the event from being. Being—especially as portrayed in his ontological system based on set theory—is marked by consistency, repetition, and indifference. The event, by contrast, is an *inconsistent multiple*, the radical excess, that cannot be derived or deduced from the situation and of which ontology can say nothing (Badiou, 2005, p. 190). It is not a fold within being, but a break with it. Thus, where Deleuze constructs a metaphysics of pure immanence—a plane in which being, becoming, and event collapse into one another—Badiou insists *on disjunction, rupture, and exception.*

Badiou radicalizes this distinction by explicitly rejecting both life and death as candidates for philosophical absolutes. He notes that many philosophical traditions—from early Hegel and Heidegger to existentialist thinkers like Sartre—have posited death (or finitude more generally) as the limit concept that grants meaning to life. For Heidegger, *being-toward-death* is the existential horizon that individuates each Dasein; for Sartre, being is bound to *past-ness*, opacity, and bad faith. These thinkers, while differing in their approaches, treat death as an ontological determinant, a structuring negativity (Badiou, 2009, p. 267–268; 2015a).

Yet for Badiou, neither life nor death holds this philosophical privilege. Both remain trapped within the framework of finitude and necessity. Both are insufficient to explain how a subject *becomes* more than an instance of life or a bearer of mortality. The event, in Badiou's view, does not derive from the life-death opposition, nor does it emerge from biological or existential concerns. Rather, it emerges as an *exception*—an occurrence that breaks with the continuity of being and opens a path toward the infinite.

In this respect, Badiou's concept of truth must be read against the vitalist image of the event. Where Deleuze celebrates becoming as vibration and creation and life as ontological creativity, Badiou sees such conceptions as insufficiently rigorous—metaphysical rather than formal, expressive rather than procedural. In Badiou's formal ontology, the event introduces a qualitative difference not by intensifying life but by suspending its parameters altogether.

The logic of exception thus becomes the architecture of truth. Against the axiom of democratic materialism—*There are only bodies and languages*—Badiou introduces the supplement: *except, there are truths* (Badiou, 2009, p. 4). These truths are not properties of bodies or effects of language. They are *exceptions* to what exists, eruptions that introduce novelty into the world, and that call for a new kind of fidelity.

Every truth, in Badiou's system, requires an eventual site and a subject. The event marks a rupture; the subject is the name for the process that unfolds its consequences. Yet the subject is not an autonomous agent in the traditional humanist sense. It is, instead, a *body organized by fidelity*—a site through which the consequences of an event are enacted and extended. The subject is always a subject *of a truth*: a point of subjective construction that emerges only in and through commitment to what exceeds it.

Crucially, Badiou does not dismiss the categories of body or world. But he reconfigures them entirely. A *body*, for Badiou, is not a biological given but the configuration of terms that sustains a truth-procedure. A *world* is not a metaphysical totality but a regime of appearance—a way in which objects appear, are ordered, and counted. The event cuts into this world, and the truth that follows introduces a new logic of visibility and intensity, a new configuration of bodies and appearances (Badiou, 2009).

From this perspective, the familiar Deleuzian lexicon—body, world, life—is not rejected but strategically *displaced*. Where Deleuze sees affirmation, Badiou installs exception. Where Deleuze valorizes immanence, Badiou posits rupture. The event is not life intensified but life interrupted—and it is in this interruption that the possibility of subjectivity, and of philosophy itself, resides.

Truth, eternity, and the ethics of fidelity

For Badiou, the subject is not a metaphysical or anthropological given. It is not an identity, an individual, or a person in any conventional sense. Rather, the subject is an *effect of exception*—a consequence of an eventual rupture that reconfigures the possible. The event, as we have seen, interrupts the logic of the world and opens a space for a new truth. It is within this space that the individual—previously no more than a living body among others—is transformed into a subject, incorporated into a subjective body. This transformation is not automatic. It requires an *intervention*: an active decision to affirm the event and pursue its consequences.

Badiou contrasts this conception of the subject with that of democratic materialism, which holds that "there are only bodies and languages." Within this dominant framework, what exists are individual lives, embodied perspectives, and discursive dispositions. There are no truths, only opinions; no subjects, only individuals. The subject, as Badiou envisions it, is unintelligible within such a framework because it is not rooted in identity or representation but in a fidelity to something *inexistent* within the world as it was.

Crucially, Badiou insists that there is not one eternal Truth but a *multiplicity of truths*, each born of a singular event. He refers to this as a *Platonism of the multiple*: a reconfiguration of Platonism that retains the category of the Idea while abandoning the unity or hierarchy of truths (Badiou, 1989). Truths are infinite in number, but each is singular in its unfolding—conditioned by the event that gave rise to it. Their eternity is not given a priori, as in Cartesian rationalism or classical metaphysics, but emerges through a process of *fidelity*, a sustained commitment to unfolding the consequences of the event in time.

Thus, Badiou's *materialist dialectic* acknowledges the reality of bodies and languages but insists that these do not exhaust the real. There are also *truths*, which interrupt and exceed material determinations. And it is precisely because truths are not inscribed within the existing structure of knowledge that they must appear as an exception.

The contemporary valorization of life—particularly in the language of human rights, humanitarian intervention, and liberal ethics—is, for Badiou, not a moral advance but a symptom of philosophical regression. In this regime, *life itself* is elevated to the status of sacred object. To be alive becomes the highest value, while suffering and death are framed as the ultimate evils. But Badiou cautions that this elevation of life—this *biopolitical sanctification* of finitude—is politically complicit with state violence, global capitalism, and imperialism. War is waged in the name of life. Markets are justified by appeals to survival. Politics is reduced to the management of human suffering.

Badiou's philosophy constitutes a radical critique of this humanitarian consensus. Against the sanctification of the human, he proposes an ethics of the *inhuman* (Badiou, 2007). Not in the sense of cruelty or dehumanization, but in the sense of fidelity to a truth that exceeds biological existence. Truth does not affirm life; it interrupts it. It forces the subject to become something other than what it was—to *subtract itself* from its worldly determination and orient itself toward eternity.

This is why Badiou consistently describes the event in terms of *hazard* or *chance* (*hasard*), and why he aligns his thinking with the poetics of Stéphane Mallarmé. Mallarmé's dictum—*The infinite comes from hazard which you have denied*—encapsulates the philosophical wager at the heart of Badiou's system. The event is not the flowering of life but its disruption. It is a throw of the dice that must be affirmed, not because it affirms life, but because it opens a path toward infinity.

In *Being and Event*, and again in *Logics of Worlds*, Badiou develops this idea rigorously: hazard is not randomness, but the *non-necessity* of the event. The event cannot be deduced from the situation; it is not part of the logic of being. To encounter the event is, therefore, to encounter a radical *outside*—not a transcendental beyond, but an exception *within* the world that cannot be explained by it. This is the Mallarméan thread in Badiou's thought: the process, or site, where hazard opens a tear in the fabric of necessity, and the infinite breaks in (Badiou, 1988; Brassier, 2000a).

As *Logics of Worlds* unfolds, this confrontation with Deleuze crystallizes in a decisive chapter titled *The Event According to Deleuze*. It is here that Badiou synthesizes decades of engagement with Deleuze's philosophy, weaving together his early political critiques, his metaphysical interventions in *Deleuze: The Clamor of Being*, and his reflections in *On Life as a Name of Being* (Badiou, 1998). This chapter marks a convergence point between early and late Badiou, early and late Deleuze—a philosophical reckoning that transcends mere commentary.

In typical fashion, Badiou formalizes his critique by casting Deleuze's metaphysics into a series of axioms—a move Deleuze himself would likely resist. But this axiomatic framing allows Badiou to isolate the core assumptions of Deleuze's theory of the event and systematically contrast them with his own. Deleuze, Badiou argues, posits the event as immanent to being, as an expression of life, as a fold within the One. Badiou, by contrast, asserts the *event as subtraction*: a rupture that introduces a new truth and generates a subject.

This formal opposition is not simply technical. It marks a fundamental divergence in what philosophy is taken to be *for*. For Deleuze, philosophy affirms difference, becoming, and immanence; it is creation of concepts. For Badiou, philosophy is the orientation to *truths*, to the inhuman and eternal dimensions of subjectivation. Where Deleuze disperses the event into a continuous flow of life, Badiou insists on the event's *punctual singularity*—its rupture, its hazard, its irreducible exception.

The event in Deleuze—four axioms

At a critical juncture in *Logics of Worlds*, Badiou crystallizes his philosophical disagreement with Deleuze by presenting what he reconstructs as the axioms of Deleuze's theory of the event. This formalization is not merely rhetorical; it is part of Badiou's broader methodological approach—drawn from mathematics—of rendering philosophical positions in their axiomatic clarity so that their implications may be precisely evaluated. While Deleuze himself avoids such schematization, Badiou's reconstruction is faithful in spirit, if not in form, to the inner logic of Deleuze's thought.

The following four axioms serve, for Badiou, as the structural pillars of Deleuze's metaphysics of the event. He articulates them not to parody, but to bring them to a point of confrontation with his own theory of the event as rupture, subtraction, and truth.

Axiom 1: Unlimited-becoming becomes the event itself. (Badiou, 2009, p382)

Deleuze, Badiou argues, equates the event with unlimited becoming—a flux without origin or terminus, which Deleuze frequently identifies with life. This is not to be confused with the infinite in the Platonic or mathematical sense. Deleuze's becoming is not formally infinite but qualitatively boundless—a life in perpetual variation and differentiation. In this view, the event is not a discrete break or interruption, but an expression of life's ongoing intensification. In Badiou's terms, this amounts to a collapse of the distinction between being and event. Rather than treating the event as a rupture in the order of being, Deleuze folds it back into the immanent movement of being-as-becoming.

Axiom 2: The Event is always what has just happened, what will happen, but never what is happening. (Badiou, 2009, p382)

The second axiom locates the Deleuzian event in a temporality outside the present. Drawing on the Stoics, Deleuze situates the event in the dimension of *aion*—a time of pure becoming, where the present is merely the frontier between the past and future. The event, then, is not something that happens now but something that will have happened, a kind of retrospective actualization. In this framework, the present is hollowed out, rendered a vanishing point in the flow of time. Badiou sees this as another way in which the event is folded into a metaphysical continuity—in this case, temporal rather than ontological.

Axiom 3: The nature of the event is other than that of the actions and the passions of the body. But it results from them. (Badiou, 2009, p383)

The event is of a different nature than the actions and passions of bodies, yet it emerges from them. Here, Deleuze introduces a metaphysical structure based on the differentiation between depth and surface, bodies and events, actions and sense. While the event is not reducible to the movements of bodies, it nonetheless arises from them. This idea, which resonates with the Stoic distinction between *lekta* (the sayable) and corporeal causes, is developed in Deleuze's work as a theory of the event-surface—an incorporeal layer that nonetheless depends on bodily events. The event is thus a kind of emergent property, arising immanently from the actions of bodies but irreducible to them. Badiou finds here an ambiguity: the event is neither entirely separate from being, nor entirely reducible to it. It hovers in a metaphysical limbo—suspended between action and sense.

Axiom 4: A life is composed of the same single Event, despite all the variety of what happens to it. (Badiou, 2009, p383)

Finally, Deleuze asserts that despite the infinite variations of a life, it is composed of a single event—a core motif or refrain that gives shape to its becoming. This musical analogy—where the event functions like a theme that recurs through difference—is central to Deleuze's understanding of both individuation and ethics. The event is the style of a life, the singularity that organizes its multiple expressions. For Badiou, however, this formulation threatens to aestheticize the event, to render it a compositional element in the metaphysical harmony of life. The event becomes not a break with the world, but a modulation of its inner consistency.

The danger Badiou identifies in Deleuze's schema is that the event is ultimately subsumed under the concept of the One—whether it be the One of life, of sense, or of becoming. In this way, the event becomes the destiny of the One, the unfolding of a pre-given continuity, and thus loses its character as *rupture*. The event is no longer exceptional, but expressive. Badiou identifies this structure as theological, echoing Lacan's aphorism: *Religion is sense* (Badiou, 2009, *p. 387*). To the extent that Deleuze's event is sense itself, always participates in a metaphysical order of becoming, it risks reintroducing theological structure under the guise of post-structuralist metaphysics, absorbing the event back into the One or Life (Badiou, 2009, *p. 387*).

For Badiou, the event must be thought *outside the One.* It must be conceived not as an intensification of being, but as a break from it. The event is not the culmination of becoming, but its interruption. It is this capacity for interruption—for subtracting itself from the logic of the world—that makes the event the origin of truth. And truth, in Badiou's system, does not belong to the order of sense. It is, rather, what *disrupts* the order of sense, what calls the subject into being through a fidelity to the consequences of a rupture.

To be clear, Badiou does not dismiss Deleuze's stance as a mere ideological foil. On the contrary, he often describes Deleuze as one of his closest interlocutors—a thinker whose project is serious, rigorous, and worth confronting on its own terms. The critique Badiou offers is not a rejection, but a philosophical *challenge.* He acknowledges Deleuze's achievement in breaking with classical metaphysics, particularly its metaphysics of presence and identity. But he insists that Deleuze does not go far enough. By equating the event with life, Deleuze ultimately returns to a vision of ontological continuity—a vision, Badiou contends, that must be interrupted if philosophy is to remain true to its task. Deleuze thus becomes a mirror in which Badiou defines his own philosophical position—not in opposition to difference, multiplicity, or becoming as such, but in commitment to a concept of truth that cannot be reconciled with the One, with sense, or with the metaphysical valorization of life.

The event as a way out of binary thinking

At this stage of his critique, Badiou deepens the metaphysical stakes of the debate by confronting what he calls "the old metaphysics"—a structure of thought grounded in binary oppositions: *Essence vs. Existence*, *Subject vs. Object*, *Inside vs. Outside*, *Form vs. Matter*. These pairs all ultimately participate, Badiou argues, in a broader metaphysics of presence: a system that privileges ontological immediacy, givenness, and the fullness of being.

Badiou's target here is not simply the historical residue of classical metaphysics, but the lingering hold it continues to exert on philosophical categories—even those designed to exceed it. For both Badiou and Deleuze, the *event* is the conceptual wedge that breaks open this metaphysical enclosure. The event is neither essence nor accident, neither subjectively constituted nor objectively given. Instead, it occupies an ontologically indeterminate zone—what Badiou calls *trans-being* (Badiou, 1998). It is the site of a rupture that displaces all predetermined categories. It is not what *is*, but what *happens*, and what causes a reconfiguration of the coordinates of what is.

This is also where Badiou sees a fundamental tension in Deleuze's work: the attempt to think the event as a radical break, while preserving its immanence to life, to sense, to becoming. Deleuze, Badiou acknowledges, seeks to avoid the two dominant traps of pre-Kantian metaphysics: dogmatism and empiricism. The former turns the event into a transcendental essence, a pre-given metaphysical principle (as in certain forms of rationalism or theology); the latter collapses the event into contingency—a mere empirical accident.

Deleuze's project, then, is admirable in its ambition: to think the event *as a new beginning*, while maintaining its consistency with a metaphysics of immanence. His fidelity to the Kantian imperative—to construct a theory of the conditions of possibility of experience, without lapsing into transcendental illusion—is something Badiou recognizes and respects. Indeed, *Logics of Worlds* is marked by a serious, though often implicit, engagement with Kant. Particularly in its rethinking of the object, the book gestures toward a post-Kantian transformation of objectivity (Meillassoux, 2014).

Badiou suggests that what we still lack is a fully developed post-Kantian theory of the object that detaches the object from its subordination to the subject. Deleuze, for his part, attempts precisely this: to articulate a theory of the event and the object beyond subjectivist correlation. And yet, despite this shared ambition, Badiou argues that Deleuze falls into the very metaphysical errors he seeks to overcome.

As Badiou writes (with his characteristic irony), "There's nothing to add."—"Except, that" (2009, p. 387): when Deleuze describes the event in terms of intensities, virtuality, and the unbounded continuity of becoming, he leans toward empiricism. The event becomes a function of affective intensities and differential flows—tied to lived experience, and hence caught within the flux of phenomenality. But, conversely, when Deleuze describes the event as the eternal return of difference, or as a modulation of the virtual that is always already there—that is, when he roots the event in the One of Being or Sense—he leans toward dogmatism. The event begins to resemble a metaphysical principle, an ontological constant.

Thus, despite his intentions, Deleuze ends up caught in the very binary he seeks to escape. The event oscillates between the poles of empiricism and dogmatism—as either an empirical variation of intensities or a transcendental unfolding of Being. The event, Badiou insists, must be thought neither as empirical emergence nor as ontological fullness, but as subtractive rupture: a break from the situation, a moment of exception that reorganizes the space of the possible.

This move is what allows Badiou to claim a position neither of transcendence nor immanence, but of trans-being—a non-place within the ontological regime that marks the appearance of a truth. Here, Badiou's notion of the event becomes radically anti-metaphysical, or as he says, a "metaphysics without metaphysics" (Badiou, 2000b). The event is not grounded in being, nor the truth of being, but in what breaks with being. It is not prefigured in the virtual, but *appears only to vanish,* only through an unpredictable moment of interruption—an exception without precedent.

This is also the basis for Badiou's critique of contemporary humanism and its ideological avatars. The metaphysical sanctification of "life"—often articulated through the discourse of human rights, biopolitics, or liberal humanitarianism—is, for Badiou, part of the doctrine of *democratic materialism*. By equating truth with the affirmation of life, this worldview reduces the human to a biological species and truth to opinion. What is lost is the dimension of the inexistent and the generic, the part that does not count, the element that is subtracted from or unrepresented in the state of the situation—the very condition for the emergence of a truth.

For Badiou, then, the event is the name for the possibility of a thought beyond the world—and beyond the metaphysics that structures our relation to the world. It opens a space for truth, for subjectivation, and ultimately for a different conception of life—one not reducible to survival, identity, or function, but organized around a fidelity to what interrupts the given and compels a new way of living.

Badiou's four counter-axioms

In direct response to the Deleuzian schema of the event, Badiou formulates his own four axioms—each designed to negate or invert the structure of Deleuze's metaphysical commitment to becoming, life, and continuity. What emerges is not simply a disagreement over terms, but a deep philosophical antagonism regarding the nature of rupture, temporality, embodiment, and subjectivation.

Axiom 1: The event is not the condensation of vital or immanent becoming; it is a cut in becoming.

The event introduces a break, a cut—a moment in which what was previously inexistent becomes suddenly, abruptly, maximally existent.

Axiom 2: The event is not the unity of past and future—but a separation from both.

Where Deleuze conceives the event as a temporal fold, synthesizing past and future in a musical or cinematic flow (as seen in his readings of Nietzsche and the Stoics), Badiou radically repositions the temporal function of the event. The event, for him, does not harmonize time; it dislocates it. It interrupts temporal continuity, suspends historical sequence, and inaugurates a new ordering of the present. In Badiou's terms, it creates a *new time*

Axiom 3: The event does not result from the actions or passions of bodies—it creates a new body.

The event is not of the body, and it does not arise from any pre-existing structure of affect or action. Rather, it is a supplement to being, and it produces its own subject-body in fidelity to the truth it inaugurates. This is a body constructed not through nature, instinct, or affect, but through subjective consistency over time—a body formed through discipline, intervention, and fidelity. It is, in other words, a post-evental body, organized not by its capacities but by its commitment, which often exceed these very capacities.

Axiom 4: The event is not a composition (musical or otherwise)

For Badiou =the event is not a compositional moment within a life but a dividing incision. It does not unify a life; it restructures it entirely. The event does not arrange motifs—it breaks them apart. There is no return, no harmony, no artistic recomposition. There is only the construction of a subject out of what was formerly impossible.

These four axioms constitute a complete inversion of the Deleuzian metaphysics of the event. Where Deleuze sees continuity, expression, and difference, Badiou posits rupture, interruption, and fidelity. Where Deleuze affirms a musical unfolding, Badiou insists on a discontinuous intervention.

At the heart of this disagreement lies the fundamental question of the event's relation to Being. As we have seen, for Badiou, Deleuze, despite all of his efforts to escape metaphysical dogmatism, still posits a continuity between event and being—especially through his concept of the One, or univocity, which underwrites all multiplicities, differences, and expressions (Badiou, 1997a). For Badiou, this is the moment at which Deleuze's system falls back into theological structure, or as he calls it, a "latent religiosity" (Badiou, 2019, p. 387). It reintroduces a form of sense—of ontological harmony—that Badiou, drawing on Lacan, identifies as religion.

Badiou's alternative is a militant subtraction from sense. The event is not a moment of expressive affirmation, but a gap—the unthinkable that becomes thinkable, the supernumerary supplement that defies the world's count. It is a hazard, and it is only through the slow work of fidelity—the construction of a subject body that holds to this hazard—that a truth becomes thinkable, transmissible, and active. Thus, Badiou's counter-axioms offer not only a critique of Deleuze but also a redefinition of what philosophy must do: to think rupture rather than continuity, to affirm the rare rather than the vital, and to wager truth on the inhuman exception, not the human experience of becoming

> To break with empiricism is to think the event as the advent of what subtracts itself from all experience: the ontologically un-founded and the transcendentally discontinuous. To break with dogmatism is to remove the event from the ascendancy of the One. It is to subtract it from Life in order to deliver it to the stars.
>
> (Badiou, 2009, p. 387)

Epilogue: "What is to live?"

In the final pages of *Logics of Worlds*, Badiou stages a confrontation with the question of life—no longer as a biological or affective fact, nor as an expressive force, but as a philosophical construction that must be rethought in light of the event. The title of the epilogue, "What is to Live?", echoes both revolutionary slogans and existential demands, but Badiou reconfigures the question entirely. What is it *to live*, when "life" can no longer be anchored in the ideologies of experience, expression, or humanist self-care? What does it mean to live, when to live is no longer synonymous with *surviving, thriving,* or *being oneself?*

The propositions outlined form a kind of counter-humanist ethics, a subtractive ontology of life in which life is not a given, but a consequence. They form, together, a profound response to vitalism, democratic materialism, and the metaphysical worship of "life" as value, or, in a Nietzschean manner, as the value which cannot be valued. In their place, Badiou installs an idea of life as the subjectivation of truth—not as a state or affect, but as a task, or later, as *work* (Badiou, 2018).

1. Life as eventual trace

   Life is not something that finds itself in a world, or which unfolds organically within it. Life begins with an eventual trace—that is, with the appearance of a vanishing point that punctures the fabric of the world and opens it to truth. Life, then, is not a continuity with what is, but a consequence of a break.
2. Life as presentification

   To live is to create the present—not to inhabit it passively. Badiou reclaims the category of the present from phenomenology and gives it a new content: the subjective labor of building a present that is unprecedented, unjustified, and in excess of the situation. Life is not being-there in the present, but the creation of a new present.

3 Life and the tonality of a world

Worlds are not neutral backgrounds. They have a tonality—an affective and ontological openness or closure to the event. Life is the inscription of a point, a site where the event's consequences begin to take hold. It is a punctual genesis, not a flow, and every such point is the beginning of a new world, or at least of a new logic within the world.

4 Life as subjectivation

Life is not a category of biology, identity, or agency, but a *subjective* category: to live is to be incorporated into the consequences of an event, to become a subject to a truth. And this subjectivity is not the Cartesian subject of science, nor the Nietzschean subject of forces (Deleuze, 2014), but a subject constructed through fidelity—a term Badiou reclaims from religious and political discourse alike (Badiou, 2015b).

5 The present as the being-there of eternity

Here Badiou is at his most provocative: to live is to create the being-there of eternity. Not to touch the eternal in a mystical sense, but to produce it—to bring about its presence in the form of an immortal truth within a finite world. This is the full reversal of traditional metaphysics: eternity is not that which precedes life; it is what is created in and through it, through the labor of the subject faithful to a truth. "A faithful subject creates the present as the being-there of eternity".

6 Life is not lived experience

Against the culture of experience and the valorization of embodiment and identity, Badiou asserts: life is not lived experience. It is not affect, not expression, not identity. It is an interruption of identity—a break with what is already known and lived. A life is not what is felt or expressed, but what is constructed through fidelity to an exception.

7 Against the humanism of "Live Without Ideas"

Democratic materialism, Badiou claims, offers a morality of survival: respect life, preserve life, live without truths or transcendence. It is the ideology of the culturalist and the relativist, the rights discourse, the humanitarian. Against this, Badiou insists that life without ideas is nothing. The true dignity of life is found only in its incorporation into a truth. Not life for its own sake, but life raised to the power of thought.

8 The logic of exception

Against the atonality of contemporary life, its lack of intensity or rupture, the "except" of truths (there are only bodies and languages, except that there are truths) names the chance of a new form of life. It is inhuman, not because it denies the human, but because it names what in the human is beyond the human, an exception to the human: the capacity to be seized by something greater than survival. It is not by chance that Badiou refers here to Grace (Badiou, 2008, p. 512; 1997b).

9 Truth as the rupture with all previous possibilities

> Truth is the rupture with all previous possibilities, and therefore life, as the subjective construction of truth, is a break with everything that has come before. The human is not a being of continuity, but a being of interruption—of fidelity to that which had no place. A body is the subjective appearance of a truth—a truth that is eternal precisely because it is created. And a truth is, first of all, a rupture with all previously established domains of knowledge.

In the epilogue of *Logics of Worlds*, Badiou poses once more the question that has haunted the entire work: "What is it to live?" Yet, as I have tried to show, this move is not a return to vitalism, but a provocation. To live, for Badiou, is to be capable of affirming the consequences of a truth. It is to participate, as a subject, in the unfolding of that which exceeds the given. It is not to cling to survival, to identity, or to the comfort of recognition, but to be transformed—and to remain faithful to that transformation. And yet, this fidelity is sometimes almost the same with abandonment. Abandoning what one was, exile; "loving what you will never believe twice" (Badiou, 1982, p. 339).

Badiou's thought returns philosophy to its ancient task: not the management of life, but the orientation toward the good—now redefined as the infinite consequences of a truth (Badiou, 2012a). His Platonism is neither nostalgic nor reactionary. It is a formal structure through which a contemporary subject might resist the nihilism of democratic materialism and reassert the possibility of a life oriented by something other than mere existence.

Against the backdrop of a world in which "life" is celebrated as the highest good—in biopolitical governance, humanitarian warfare, and ethical consumerism—Badiou's philosophy stages a rupture. It invites us to conceive of life not as a value in itself, but as the site of possible exception. To live, then, is not simply to persist or to flourish. It is to affirm the consequences of that which, in interrupting life, gives it its only real value. Badiou's work does not ask us to reject life. It asks us to subtract ourselves from its dominant logic—to encounter the event, to remain faithful to its consequences, and, in doing so, to become subjects of a truth. It is this fidelity, discipline and the "heroism of existing in the affirmative joy which is universally generated by following consequences through", and not survival, that defines the ethics of living in truth (Badiou, 2009, p. 514).

What does it mean, then, to live? Not to persist. Not to flourish. Not to survive. Not to express oneself. Neither to abide by the animal, nor to dwell in its habitual abode. But to construct fidelity in the wake of a rupture, to bear the exception, and to produce eternity in time. To make the present present, not as presence, but as the appearance of a truth. It names a life not governed by the organic, nor by affect, nor by the state—but by the hazardous and perilous, immortal work of a truth. And so, in place of life as given, Badiou gives us life as a task. A subject is not born, nor found, nor expressed. A subject is constructed, and life, in its truest form, is this construction. To live, then, is to bring into the world that which the world cannot contain—and to remain faithful to it. To be present in the present. To create the being-there of eternity, "here and now, already and forever" (Badiou, 1987).

Bibliography

Badiou, Alain. (1982) *Théorie du Sujet.* Paris: Éditions Seuil.

Badiou, Alain. (1987) *Un Soirée Philosophique*. Paris: Éditions Potemkine.

Badiou, Alain. (1988) *L'Être et l'Événement.* Paris: Éditions Seuil.

Badiou, Alain. (1989) *Manifeste pour la Philosophie*. Paris: Éditions Seuil.

Badiou, Alain. (1997a) *Deleuze. La Clameur de l'Être.* Paris: Hachette Littératures.

Badiou, Alain. (1997b) *St. Paul. La Fondation d'Universalisme.* Paris: PUF.

Badiou, Alain. (1998) *Court Traité d'Ontologie Transitoire.* Paris: Éditions Seuil.

Badiou, Alain. (1999) *Conditions*. Paris: Éditions Seuil.

Badiou, Alain. (2000a) 'Un, multiple, multiplicité(s).' in *Multitudes,* vol. 1 no, 1, 195–211.

Badiou, Alain. (2000b) 'Metaphysics and the critique of Metaphysics.' Translated by A. Toscano. *In Pli: The Warwick Journal of Philosophy,* no, 10, 174–190.

Badiou, Alain. (2005) *Being and Event*. Translated by O. Feltham. London: Continuum.

Badiou, Alain. (2007) *The Century*. Translated by A. Toscano. Cambridge/Malden, MA: Polity Press.

Badiou, Alain. (2008) *Logiques des Mondes. L'Être et l'Événement II.* Paris: Éditions Seuil.

Badiou, Alain. (2009) *Logics of Worlds. Being and Event II.* Translated by A. Toscano. London: Continuum.

Badiou, Alain. (2012a) *La République de Platon.* Paris: Fayard.

Badiou, Alain. (2012b) *The Adventure of French Philosophy*. Translated by B. Bosteels. London: Verso.

Badiou, Alain. (2015a) *Le Séminaire. Nietzsche: L'Antiphilosophie I (1992–1993)*. Paris: Fayard.

Badiou, Alain. (2015b) 'Down with Death' στο Verso books blog, 18/8/2015: https://www.versobooks.com/blogs/2176-badiou-down-with-death. Last viewed 19/10/2023.

Badiou, Alain. (2018) *Immanence des Vérités.* Paris: Fayard.

Brassier Ray. (2000) 'Stellar Void or Cosmic Animal? Badiou and Deleuze on the Dice-Throw.' in *Pli: The Warwick Journal of Philosophy,* no. 10, 200–216.

Deleuze, Gilles. (1969) *Logique du Sens*. Paris: Éditions de Minuit.

Deleuze, Gilles. (2014) *Nietzsche et la Philosophie.* Paris: Presses Universitaires de France.

Kamecke, Gernot. (2009) 'What is to Live? Critical Considerations with Regard to Badiou and Bergson concerning Life Theory and Language' in *Filozofski Vestnik,* vol. xxx, no. 2, 207–225.

Meillassoux, Quentin. (2014) 'Decision and Undecidability in *Being and Event I* and *II*'. In *Parrhesia,* vol. 19, 22–35.

Chapter 12

The Unborn rags of the mind

Richard Barker

Introduction

Affect theory and Buddhism make interesting companions and lend theoretical expansion/contraction and experiential substance when applied to the sometimes stale world of psychotherapy and counselling. The latter can become neatly boxed and lacks the radical depth of Buddhism and affect theory as expressed by Brian Massumi. As poetry lies at the heart of some of the most subversive philosophy (Spinoza, Nietzsche, Deleuze and Guattari, Derrida, Laplanche, Massumi), so the metaphor of the 2,500-year-old Buddhist *kesa* provides a historical precursor and teaching which, when intimately understood, strips away any possibility of a finite, closed system of knowledge which serves to limit and imprison.

Metaphors simmer with suggestions. So too, the garments of a Zen priest. The *hossu* (fly whisk), the begging bowl, the circle and lotus hook of the kesa, the walking staff with its three rings, and even the bold head of the monk, all redolent with surprise when seen for the first time and used as teaching aids to deepen a *becoming* understanding over time.

This chapter will look at the metaphor of the kesa and place it within one area of affect theory, in order to expand psychotherapy and prevent its decline into leaden pathology.

The Kesa

The Zen monk's full kesa, worn for meditation and ceremonies, is modelled on the robe worn by the historical Buddha, Shakyamuni. It is a simple one-piece garment made of a patchwork design, covering most of the body, and draped over the left shoulder.

The original instructions for making the kesa specified that only discarded fabric—*pāmsudā*—could be used. For example, cloth that has been burned by fire, munched by oxen, gnawed by mice, worn by the dead, a menstruation rag, or an "excrement sweeping cloth"—*funzoe* in Japanese ("Tibet House US Cultural Center of H.H. The Dalai Lama," 2021, para. 1). These rags were then washed, purified, and sewn into a kesa.

DOI: 10.4324/9781003669906-13

Later the robe was made from fabric presented by lay devotees. Overtime, as Buddhist teachings became more mainstream and accepted by society, the merchants and wealthy would present materials, such as silks woven with gold brocade. Twenty years into his ministry, the Buddha formalised the patchwork pattern in the monastic rules as follows:

> Once too when the Blessed One was on His way home from Rajagaha to the Southern hills, He said to the venerable Ananda [his disciple attendant or chaplain]:
>
> "Ananda, do you see the land of Magadha laid out in squares, laid out in strips, laid out with borders, laid out with crosslines?"
>
> "Yes, Lord."
>
> "Try to arrange robes for bhikkhus [monks] like that, Ananda."
>
> (Hollenbeck, 2010, p. 2)

The "squares" the Buddha referred to were rice paddy fields. So the pattern of the rice fields was woven into the monks' clothing.

Hence, the original practical and spiritual interdependence of monastics and laity: the monks depended on the farmers and lay devotees for their food and the monks gave their teaching (*Dharma*) in return.

The humble origins of the kesa were not forgotten and are implicit in the teaching of Buddhist practice. For example, we can see the First Noble Truth, *There Is Suffering*, mirrored in the discarded and rejected, bloodied, and refused rags used to make the original kesa: a psychological parallel of disturbance which may exist on the edge of consciousness or is not seen at all. A disturbance that we turn away from and remains hidden but is actually the very manure and compost of our lives. If we return and remember, and dip our feet in the river, we may yet feel its current and get to know a different, unknowable, unborn teacher.

When a nun places the kesa on her head after morning meditation, she recites: "How great and wondrous are the clothes of enlightenment, formless and embracing every treasure. I wish to unfold the Buddha's teaching that I may help all living beings" (Jiyū-Kennett, 1993a, The Order of Buddhist Contemplatives, p. 14).

The "formless", as mentioned above, is sometimes called the Unborn.

The Unborn and affect theory

Perhaps there may be a linguistic equivalent of the Unborn in affect theory. According to Massumi (2019):

> Specifically in relation to language … there is an unabsorbed remainder of meaning left over after the statement is said and done. This is meaning that has yet to come to determinate expression, so it is, strictly speaking, nonsense. But is not nonsense simply as the opposite of sense. It is nonsense as a surplus of sense, brewing with meanings to come. It is what Guattari, following Hjelmslev, sometimes calls "purport"—pure matter of meaning, as yet syntactically and

> semantically unformed, but already pragmatically preaccelerated (…) Significations and propositions in the conventional logical sense try to capture affective intensity, and fail. Affect is always already elsewhere before the last "i" is dotted.
>
> (pp. 114–15)

Hence, affect is autonomous. So too a common meditation experience of the Unborn: a powerful somatic, unabsorbed, a surplus of sense, becoming, yet to come.

In the Heart Sutra of Mahayana Buddhism, monks sing of this insight, "No eye, ear, nose, tongue, sound, colour, touch or objects (…) always becoming" (Jiyū-Kennett, 1993a, p. 34).

For Massumi (2019), there is a place where "rationality has to learn to be a catalyst, instead of a sovereign" (p. 118). Similarly, in Buddhism, there is no sovereign. Any affect or experience has its death implanted: all things are passing.

So too the Unborn is not sovereign—not transcendent—as it needs to be expressed here, now. There is an impersonal relationship with the personal. The Unborn needs form, although form cannot fully express it. It will remain hidden and autonomous—"a permanent periphery" (Wayne Matthews, personal communication, 2024). And as this autonomy is expressed, it will die. You cannot capture affective intensity. It is already "elsewhere".

This nonsovereign emptiness is inherent and exterior to the individual who becomes less than, or perhaps as stated by Massumi (2019), "transindividual" (p. 116).

To understand this, bowing is necessary: modesty and humility are necessary. We align with the arrows of a compass in mind and heart which point to the parts and rags that make up the kesa. We may visit one section of the field, one place of intensity, suffering, and transformation, but there is always another. Another place of darkness and Unborn potential, and each refers to the other, each one bows. We are known and unknown in emptiness.

Some of these rags of the kesa come together, just for a while: a becoming and stitching together. At this point, we may perceive a sentient, conscious person, animal, insect, a tree—an awakening, an insight. Just for a while, there is a square earth-bound mandala, a kesa, until the field and person are consumed, and the husks of rice become the compost of a new lotus flower.

The activity and becoming of this Unborn is tantalisingly close to Artaud's idea of the "body without organs" and the Autonomy of Affect of Massumi.

As for the not born, so it would seem for Massumi that affects precede emotional states. There is a latent lack in our knowledge of what we experience: an unknown. Massumi (2023) states that "Affect is not a personal feeling (…) Affect is a non-conscious experience of intensity" (Waller, 2023, par. 13).

This non-conscious intensity of experience is not unlike the visceral experience of the Unborn and its compassion: a bringing to deeper awareness and intensity of the sometimes rotten karmic rags that have become the trainee's knotted emotions.

This takes time to unfold.

These rags are unseen *and* experienced sometimes as suffering and disturbance. It is very hard and often unnecessary to know where this disturbance comes from, but it is essential to sit within the heart of it. It can feel unknown, awkward, and unwanted. Like the suffering kesa rags of the nun who transforms them into the clothes of enlightenment.

It is her sewing together of the kesa, paralleled in the acceptance and embrace of these disparate rejected rags of self and other, which may bring together and unfold understanding and awareness over the nun's lifetime.

The Kesa as a representation of the precepts

A traditional view of the kesa is that it represents the precepts, which are teachings of how to live skilfully, passed down to the disciple from the deep understanding (*kensho*/enlightenment) of a Zen master.

The rags, living via the precepts, and enlightenment are seen as the same thing but must be fully absorbed to be understood as such.

Hence, the bodily intimacy and embrace of the nun who literally unfolds these precepts and suffering rags and wraps them around herself.

In this way, she takes refuge within the Unborn: a lotus flower cannot kill. She has taken refuge in the precepts.

These rags of life have been affected across a fabric of other bodies unseen: transindividual, unconscious, in the body intensities, in unholy conversation from time immemorial, and now the nun, having sewn them together, will attempt to make sense of them by letting go of them.

As Dōgen (2007) wrote:

> When one studies Buddhism, one studies oneself, when one studies oneself, one forgets oneself, when one forgets oneself one is enlightened by everything, and this very enlightenment breaks the bonds of clinging to both body and mind, not only for oneself but for all beings as well.
>
> (p. 206)

Just so, she wraps the rice paddy field around her. The whole earth becomes her refuge as she disappears into the Unborn and the sanctuary of the alterity of affects.

From unconditioned Unborn and without organs to conditioned body of refused, karmically charged rags. Of these rags, which covered and absorbed the blood and excrement of others and of the land, she slowly, patiently makes a mandala flower. The affect of these rags brings help to those she prays with, seen and unseen, and all returns to the Unborn.

She has no idea what this seemingly autonomous other is but guards it well, or else all is lost, and so begins a hell realm of nonsense.

The affective therapeutic encounter

The therapist will often visit this hell realm with his or her client.

In therapy, perhaps you and I—counsellor and client—are like the nun: far more than just these two. We are transindividual and come from the rags and the stench of the compost of many. We are imagined from a place of not knowing and invisible, non-conscious visceral intensities. Just for a while, the many affects of what is said and not said—evoked, suggested, felt in a change of temperature or atmosphere, and the felt texture of it, helpfully distracted by the weight of a passing comment or disturbing metaphor, which necessarily allays and helps the client forget an initial concern, which plummets the meeting to new depth, like the discordant rags of the *kāṣāya*—may be sewn together. Via Unborn exchange of speech and otherwise, a helpful turn of phrase or intervention may then be expressed before the autonomy of affect makes us thankfully lost for words again.

Indeed, it helps to forget the self. And silence is important.

Here we may feel discomfort in the room, or perhaps some peace.

As Massumi (2019) stated: "As with the autonomy of affects, meaning is as much in the gaps between the words as in the words themselves" (p. 115).

As the Buddha said, look outside the squares of the rice paddy field; see the fields become visible by the "strips, laid out with borders, laid out with crosslines" (Hollenbeck, 2010, p. 2).

Alongside the rags of the *kāṣāya* is silence.

When the therapeutic encounter encourages silence—when we maybe helpfully forget what we wanted to say for a moment—a gap, a void appears, and we may be disturbed. To the point, we may want to rush in and fill it. But let that gap speak for a while, feel the disturbance, and let the forgotten rags sing an unholy thought. Just the lip and curl of it is enough.

And then, as in art, when your eyes are deflected from the scrap and rash of the born image and meaning is sensed, so in therapy, when there is a virtual movement which spins off from the initial spoken words, and instead there is a felt, visceral, on-the-skin perception and cognition, then you are feeling the affective force of it. A moment of insight and enlightenment may arise.

The female monastic Rev. Master Jiyū (1993b) identifies wearing the kesa of the Unborn with her reason for living and says, just before she is given the Buddhist precepts:

> My purpose for living is to be a monk (…) I have been a monk for many years but—what *is* a monk? My kesa is upon my head and the Lord of the House, That Which Is, pulls its corner. Yes, indeed, this *is* monkhood—to wear the kesa of the Lord; true ordination is to *know* what it is to be a monk.
>
> (p. 25)

In the intimacy of a therapeutic encounter, something, or someone, pulls at a corner of the scraps of affects; the lip and barnacled curl of it. The rest remains unseen, autonomous though implicit, in the intensity of perception of this unassertive wave and urgent scrap of life. Something pulls at a corner when the urgency promotes itself and the discarded and homeless becomes the whole of enlightenment and we are seen.

Just for a while, we understand.

This will carry a conceptually complex movement of thought and feeling that wants nothing more than to keep generating more concepts and affects, beyond where the author, the homeless monk, the transindividual counsellor/client's insight stopped.

There is an affective potency and generative conversation, which has come from the rags of the Unborn—from nowhere—which moves towards the surplus … of always having more to say than knowing how to say it.

Trusting in this abundance, in these rags, we take a risk and jump. We transform the forgotten suffering, stitch it together, and feel the affect of love.

Bibliography

Aemilius. (2010, March). Tradition of the Buddhist robe. *The Dharma Wheel,* para. 1. https://www.dharmawheel.net/viewtopic.php?t=17625

Benjamin, B.S. (2002). Historical Buddhist *kesa* robes as inspiration for contemporary fiber art. *Silk Roads, Other Roads: Textile Society of America 8th Biennial Symposium,* p. 389. https://digitalcommons.unl.edu/tsaconf/503/

Hollenbeck, O. (2010). The Buddhist kesa: Clothes of enlightenment. *Terebess,* p 2. https://terebess.hu/zen/szoto/kesa.pdf

Massumi, et al. (2019). Affect and Immediation: An interview with Brian Massumi. *Disclosure: A Journal of Social Theory, 28* (13), 114–116, 118. https://doi.org/10.13023/disclosure.28.09

Śūnyatā. (2024, November 17). In *Wikipedia.* https://en.wikipedia.org/wiki/Śūnyatā

Tibet House US Cultural Center of H.H. The Dalai Lama. (2021). https://thus.org/whats-in-a-robe/#:~:text=The%20Japanese%20equivalent%20of%20pāmsūda,around%20and%20cover%20the%20mendicant

Rev. Master Jiyū-Kennett, P.T.N.H. (Ed.) (1993a). *The monastic office.* (1st ed.). Shasta Abbey Press.

Rev. Master Jiyū-Kennett, P.T.N.H. (Ed.) (1993b). *How to grow a lotus blossom or how a Zen Buddhist prepares for death* (2nd ed.). Shasta Abbey Press.

Rev. Master Jiyū-Kennet, P.T.N.H. (Ed.) (2007). *Zen is eternal life.* Shasta Abbey Press.

Waller, L., Introduction to affect Theory: Brian Massumi & Eve Sedgwick. Then & Now. https://www.thenandnow.co/2023/06/15/introduction-to-affect-theory-brian-massumi-eve-sedgwick/#:~:text=Affects%20are%20a%20way%20of,-conscious%20experience%20of%20intensi retrieved 2023, June 24

Chapter 13

"Have you ever found yourselves *in sense?*"

On pathos and affect

Nikolaos Kypriotakis

Pathos – bodily felt and expressed, fluid, ever-evolving and context-dependent – referred to a broad spectrum of pre-reflective experience: from a subtle sense of unease to the capacity for suffering, to powerful, intense emotions, feelings, or illness, incidental or qualitative change, etc. (Its verbal cognate *paschein* means to suffer).

Sense – as pre-conceptual, pre-reflexive, bodily sense of life and situations, as raw (before conceptualizations) feeling and responsive energy – can be seen as affect, while affectivity can be conceptualized as the capacity to experience affect and the ongoing process of experiencing, acting and meaning-making.

What does it mean for us to be conscious *in sense*? To cross the threshold of an event or situation and enter the implicit intricacy and unseparated multiplicity, into the emergent relational, valuing field of language, concern, potentialities, prehensions and abductions, mutual intertwinement and becoming?

Thinking and feeling in a life-affirmative way (bodily, immersively, affectively, *in sense* and with pathos) might need a kind of co-capacitation, or transindividual relation (in education, in therapy, etc.). But how? And why?

Have you ever *found* yourself *in sense*? Inside *emotion, sensation*, in *pathos*, into *feeling*? Have you ever *found* yourself in the exhausting triumph of the senses?

In loving-dying delirium, incensed? In any kind of supra-affecting-affective-affected, highly and deeply sensible/sensitive state? A transitory, liminal process of movement and natality, where the boundaries between inner and outer are blurred, in a mess of chaotic, extreme arousal, of death and rebirth, where the habitual words and meanings lose their usual significance, while still functioning into the bristling moments of vitality? A kind of non-reversible, immediate transition beyond the usual semantic referents, but all the more visionary and even painful, vibrant and expansive?

What is it with *affect*, *pathos* and *sense* or any kind of *liminality*?

Felt body

According to Hermann Schmitz (2023), a paradigm shift occurred in Greece around the 2nd half of the 5th century B.C., a kind of "psychologistic-reductionistic-introjectionist objectification of reflection (*Besinnung*)", that "both Christianity

DOI: 10.4324/9781003669906-14

and the natural sciences took advantage of" and which was "brought to far-reaching success in the following century by Plato and Aristotle" (p. 28). A division of the world occurred; a thin slice of the world (now the bounded) "soul" or "psyche" was assigned to every conscious being as a kind of private, inner world of introjected, lived experience. Feelings and emotions began to be perceived as introjected, and private as well as "*passiones animae*, affects or passions of the soul" (p. 37). This constituted one of the "great losses of important dimensions of normal life experience" (p. 28), along with the splitting into physical body (*Körper*) and soul. The same destiny of disappearance (as our focal point), oblivion and repression has befallen upon our sensed, felt body (*Leib*), to feelings as atmospheres and to our felt-bodily affective communication and involvement in the world, to surface-less spaces in general (along with the surface-containing spaces of geometry), to the studying of situations with an internally diffused significance, to felt-bodily islands (instead of organs of the senses, for example), etc.

In the *Iliad*, we can find an example of a not purely psychic view of human experience; everything, counter to Modernity, is explained upon "felt-bodily impulses and not the differentiation of the organs of sense", while in the *Odyssey*, things have already changed. This kind of archaic felt-bodily dynamism can also be found in certain specific characteristics of Pythagoreans, in Empedocles, Aeschylus (as contrasted to Sophocles), Heraclitus, in the Stoics and even in St Paul, etc. (Griffero in Schmitz, 2019; Griffero, 2024, pp. 18–19).

When Schmitz (2023, p. 33) writes about the human felt body and feelings as atmospheres, he is referring to:

> the incarnation of everything that one can feel oneself and as belonging to oneself, around, but not always inside one's physical body, without relying on the five senses of sight, hearing, touch, smell, and taste, or on the perceptive schema built on their perception.

A crucial concept: feeling

Allocating *feeling* (also) to the social/cultural and material/environmental (in unity), and not (only) to some kind of personal place, or to individual psychology, subverts the usual tendencies of separating the personal/individual and the social, the inner and the outer, or even the affective from the rational.

Aware of such separation is also Raymond Williams (1977) via his concept of embryonic-phase, practical mode(s) of consciousness, called structures of feeling/experience, or forming/formative processes, at the edge of semantic availability, distinct from other precipitated, social semantic formations or formed wholes from the past.

Along with feeling, affect is also one of the definitive psychological categories together with experience, self, subjectivity, desire, body etc., to name a few. What is more, terms such as feeling, pathos, passion, affect, emotion, mood and sensation, share a long and entangled history regarding their emergence, their use and their differentiated meanings.

According to Dixon (2003), "the current concept of 'emotion' only emerged in English around 1800 (a little earlier in French), supplanting near synonymous terms like 'passions', 'sentiments' and 'affections' generally used prior to that point" (Richards & Stenner, 2023, p. 124).

It is remarkable that within the history of English-language psychological thought, the decades between 1800 and 1850 saw the emergence of a wholesale change in established vocabulary related to theoretical discussions about phenomena such as hope, fear, love, hate, joy, sorrow, anger no longer primarily discussed as passions or affections of the soul but almost invariably referred to as "the emotions" (Dixon, 2003, p. 4).

In his introduction to the English translation of Auerbach's classic philological essay *Passio as Passion*, Elsky (2001) reminds us that "the history of the changing contents of a word reflects the changing values of a culture": how did the ancient Greek term 'passive' (*pathos*, "suffering/affliction") – rendered as *passio* by the Stoics, through its early Christian, passion mysticism and medieval transformations and understandings – could reach the full unfolding of its meaning over the competing expression *affectus*, as *passions* [*Leidenschaften*] and then as feeling (*Gefühl*), sensation (*Empfindung*)?

Although in Aristotelian dialectics, according to Auerbach (1941), psychic *pathos* can be considered a movement of the soul and potentiality, *pathos-passio* is related to the verb *paskhô/paschein)* (to suffer, experience or to be affected) (Konstan, 2006).

Although "affect" may be used as an overarching term – or a generic, categorical and metapsychological term, not descriptive of a specific referent (Green, 1977; Stenner, 2017) – some tend to make a more clear distinction between "affect" and "emotion": "Emotion", which often metaphorically suggests something like "internal motor", which "*moves* the organism from within" (Richards & Stenner, 2023, p. 125), may be considered a kind of more identifiable affect, while affect in general implies to affect something as much as "being affected by something" (by another body, encounters or events), directly or indirectly, consciously or pre-consciously (Hearn, 2021, p. 92). Nevertheless, many have argued against such distinctions (Hearn, 2021, p. 92; Wetherell, 2012, 2013). Reeser (2023, p. 6) writes that "the very separation between 'affect' (as non-discursive and visceral) and 'emotion' (as discursive and culturally coded) risks reifying a binarized gender split".

Stenner (2017) is one of those questioning the affect/emotion distinction, against the "affect is not emotion" view, suggesting "feeling" (the Whiteheadian, relational, process of prehending; not just a sensation but a feeler-felt relation) as a crucial concept (actually a kind of Ariadne's thread) in this conceptual puzzle (Richards & Stenner, 2023, p. 126), following very closely Spinoza's (1677/1989) central notions of encounter and power, insisting that Spinoza does not draw an affect/emotion distinction and that his thought/extension parallelism prevents any (1995, p. 88) notion of affect as "irreducibly bodily" (Massumi, 1995, p. 88).

A more general concept of Spinozian ontological affect (*affectus*/*affectio*) that encompasses all nature, all entities (not just humanity), as well as the Whiteheadian, processual concept of (physical) "feeling", in its most expanded meaning, could be for Stenner (2017) a kind of transdisciplinary synthesis of all the other, different notions of "affect":

- "affect" as a categorical, technical, scientific, psychotherapeutic, psychological, psychoanalytic, psychodynamic or psychosocial concept (e.g., "affect" and the unconscious, or the non-conscious, the drive energy, etc.) (e.g., Green, 1977; Soler, 2016),
- affect as encounter, viewed under the attribute of bodily extension,
- affect as a Spinozian, anthropological, transformative encounter,
- affect as self-creation (all entities are relationally and fundamentally composed out of "the power relations they participate within" (pp. 217–218),
- affect as virtual (Massumi, 2002), related to affect as intensity (Massumi, 1995),
- affect as in affect system theory by Silvan Tomkins (1962),
- affect as a Queer theory and cultural studies concept (Sedgwick & Frank, 1995).
- affect as two-sided, virtual/actual, liminal phenomenon (or vector, a phenomenon of liminality) of a process of transition/transference (or feeling, e.g., Whitehead, 1929/1985): "a mixed and liminal space/time of becoming 'betwixt and between' virtual and actual forms of order" (Stenner, 2017, p. 213).

Human affectivity as liminality

Anthropological affectivity, as the last item of the previous list indicates, Stenner (2017, p. 15) informs us, can be usefully conceptualized as the experience of liminality (liminal affectivity and affectivity as liminality, transformation, emergence and becoming), whether spontaneous – unstaged: events that happen to us; death(s), accidents, crises, disasters, etc. – or devised – staged, fabulated, ritualized: performative events we "do" to ourselves; "self-created through the mediation of an objectified liminal medium" (p. 104) – or any such complex mixture:

> We experience liminality when the forms of process (socio-psycho-organico-physical) that usually sustain, enable and compose our lives are, for some reason, disrupted, interrupted, transformed or suspended.
>
> (p. 14)

From van Gennep's (1909/1960) rites of passage to Turner (1969/1995, 1982) and Árpad Szakolczai (2009, 2016), liminal experiences/occasions, the "in-between moments when conventional limits are removed" (Stenner, 2017, p. 262), "tend to be highly affective in nature because they are formative moments of great significance: leaps into the unknown" (p. 15). These are the experiences that *change* us, experiences we *must go through*, at least in their liminal phases, in between the "preliminal rites of separation" and the "postliminal rites of incorporation" (pp. 15, 62), "immersed in a paradoxical logic that is *both* 'both/and' *and* 'neither/nor' ... a logic of the 'betwixt and between'" (Stenner, 2017, p. 15).

Vitality affects

Regarding different notions of affect, one should *add* to the above list, if they care about not "reducing the sense of living, vivid immediacy that is associated with 'forming processes' to the merely personal and subjective, abstracted from the material and objective" (Stenner, 2017, p. 222). For example, one may add Daniel Stern's (2010) "dynamic forms of vitality" (or "vitality affects" among other terms used for the same aspect) – what Susanne Langer (e.g., 1953) would call "forms of feeling" – what gives to content (to the "discontinuous, digital, categorical nature of words", p. 110) its movement, its basic, non-verbal, analogical, phenomenal, Gestalt/sense of being alive and dynamically flowing, "at the interface between the narrative and the physiological" (p. 37).

> [Vitality forms] unite the elements that put flesh on experience so that it is felt and seen as coming from a living person existing in our real daily world –someone who moves in time and space, and with force and direction.
>
> (Stern, 2010, p. 30)

Forms of vitality are part of the "implicit relational knowing" (and socio-affective competence, in general) in all interpersonal, inter-psychic, happenings and events (Stern, 2010, p. 111) of sharing and interchanging experience, as well as part and building blocks of the internalization processes of interactive experiences due to the "affective value" of "objects" (p. 144).

We might also include the central role of "arousal systems/functions" (Tomkins, 1962), regarding the dynamic (alive) features of experience, as well as affect attunement (vitality form matching) and affect regulation (Stern, 2010), etc.

A lot of senses seem to be involved in the sense of living, vivid immediacy, a whole sensual self (Leikert, 2019):

> the basic five senses (hearing, smelling, tasting, seeing, feeling), which are complemented by other sensual competencies, such as temperature (thermoreception), pain (nociception), balance (vestibular sense), depth (proprioception), and several interoceptions (e.g., thirst, hunger, and blood-pressure regulation), which function as detectors or sensors.
>
> (Schultz-Venrath, 2024, p. 10)

Many forms of non-verbal or body-oriented psychotherapies deal directly with such senses of living as well as affect, relying heavily and focusing on the "sense" of experience/ing, on the "feel" of its unique occurrence and situational emergence, usually under a holistic and processual perspective (i.e., Gendlin's Focusing-oriented Therapy, different kinds of Gestalt Therapies, music therapies, dance therapies, etc.), using different theoretical constructs of various levels of complexity and analysis (and fragmentations) around terms such as "body/soma", "mind", "self", "experience" and "affect".

"Sensing" and (re)searching for such different kinds of "senses" and their attributes expands to all kinds of fields of inquiry: from philosophy, physiology, psychology and psychotherapy, old and contemporary, to developmental psychology, neuroscience, neurobiology and neuropsychology, to name a few.

From the Aristotelean (*De Anima*) *sensus communis* (*koinē aisthēsis*; common feeling, a kind of universal sense, evident in all modalities), "comprising all sensual perceptions that have their origin within the organism and are not part of the usual five senses" (Schultz-Venrath, 2024, p. 9), there is a search for supra-sensory attributes and supra-modal forms, primitive sensibility/ies, pan-modal phenomena and super-Gestalt(s) of different levels of complexity, where dynamic forms of vitality (and/or affect) would just be a "force, motion, time, space and intentionality all combined" such a Gestalt (Stern, 2010, pp. 26–27), while, for example, Gendlin's (1996) felt sense/ing, felt gesture/ing and felt shift would just be considered a larger, more complex, holistic, emergent Gestalt/sense of a whole situation, where affective forms of vitality are "an important part of the whole", a lower-level Gestalt (Stern, 2010, p. 53).

New equivalents of a search for a *sensus communis* – like body self, body scheme, body image (Fuchs, 1995) – for a kind of intermodal integration/perception and action space, which is constantly forming the phenomenal world and the sensorimotor interactions with the environmental affordances, together with affective directedness and intentionality and the basic sense of self-awareness and self-affection, generally inform the "binding problem" in neuroscience (Fuchs, 2018, pp. 20, 60).

But what is crucial here is not just any kind of modernized theory-geometry but a step further, beyond just the lines of Pierre-François Moreau's comment (2003), where passion(s) can be a synonym or an envelope for affect(s).

Affect as pathos

Aristotle treats *pathê* in a detailed and systematic only way in the *Rhetoric* (Konstan, 2006, p. 38) "as responses not to events but to actions, or situations resulting from actions, that entail consequences for one's own or others' relative social standing" (p. 40), following the "classical view of *pathê* as arising primarily in and from social interactions" (p. 39), in a teleological (useful, purposeful) perspective which reminds us of functionalist and evolutionist psychology theories about emotions: pain and pleasure, suffering, grieving and rejoicing, loving and hating involved in the emotions' effect on our judgements them (Konstan, 2006, p. 34; Moreau, 2003, p. 35: "ordinary people … must … have been intensely aware of relative degrees of power and their own vulnerability to insult and injury" (Konstan, 2006, p. 259).

Nevertheless, *pathos* emerges in Aristotle's entire oeuvre, together with closely related, different grammatical forms of the term. In Aristotle and in classical Greek, *πάθος* may refer, in general, to "affective change(s)" (*Metaphysics* V.21): secondary qualities in respect of which a thing can be altered (as opposed to its essence) (potential changes); such accomplished alterations (actualized changes, qualitative changes, effects); injurious, painful alterations/movements; misfortunes, accidents, sufferings, what befalls a person, painful experiences on a large scale. Also, the neutral significance of a circumstance, incidental happenings/changes, mental activities/phenomena such as remembering, and emotions as reactions to impinging events, but mostly social transactions (Konstan, 2006, pp. 3–4; Oele, 2020, pp. 167, 186). What is more, the term *pathos* may have acquired a sense similar to that of an "emotion" around 420 CE or even later (Harris, 2001, p. 84; Konstan, 2006, p. 16).

At the beginning of *Agamemnon*, in Aeschylus' trilogy of tragedies, *Oresteia*, during the *parodos*, the entrance of the Chorus, in the "Hymn to Zeus", we hear:

> one who enthusiastically calls on Zeus with songs of victory will be wholly in his right mind – Zeus who put men on the road to wisdom, who laid down and made valid the law 'by suffering, learning'. There drips before the heart, instead of sleep, the pain that reminds of suffering; and good sense comes to one against one's will. Violent, it seems, is the favour of the gods who sit on the august bench of command.
>
> (Sommerstein, 2010, p. 122)

"violent favour", violent grace, is (*pathei mathos*), the learning by *pathos*, the learning by suffering.

This reminds us of Nietzsche's *The Birth of Tragedy*, where "suffering (*Leiden*) is part of that primal unchanging ground of reality the Dionysian spirit celebrates" and the notion of the "tragicization" of early Greek philosophy (or even tragedy's appropriation of philosophy and the Pre-Socratic and Homeric traditions); a Nietzschean life-affirming, life-denying opposition, a dialectics pro- and against a kind of Socratic rationalism and moral intellectualism, with regards to *sophroneîn*, to acquiring the grace of "good sense", "wisdom", "true knowledge" (Scapin, 2020, pp. 238–240).

This tension has never left humanity, in all its human-very-human twists and turns, through disasters and revelations: the search for "true knowledge", whatever that may be, for "divinity", even without any kind of God, in the passion of ecstasy and the completeness of pain and horror, in the most wonderful joy of life and bodies (all kinds of bodies) and in the most barbaric misery, in the divine, hyper-complex "organicity" of nature, alongside the most vibrant, anarchic principle of the vital, forceful interactivity and inter-affectivity of the elements that make up the totality of the world.

In this context of the implicit and explicit (semantic) complexity of the passages of *pathos* through antiquity, the archaic and the ancient world, to Continental Thought and secular life/love (Auerbach, 1941; Besnier, Moreau & Renault, 2003; Dixon, 2003; Konstan, 2006; Moreau & Ramond, 2006, etc.), Aristotle occupies a prominent place in this multidimensional universe. Not only for his valuable distinctions and categorizations, but mainly because he testifies to and records the echoes of earlier, concepts, rituals and religious traditions, setting directions beyond those of analytical thinking, giving a sense of the breadth and depth of this concept, its multitude of dimensions in philosophical thought, political and community life, the arts, ethics, etc., together with all the additions, counterpositions, expansions, etc.

Following such passages of *pathos*, Buch (2010, p. 20) comments that:

> [T]he term *pathos* seems to have a remarkable capacity to span opposites: external and internal, trigger and reaction, spontaneous affect and reflective distance, being overpowered and asserting oneself anyway, instinctive compassion and staged emotionality, the grandeur of suffering and the recognition of its futility. The modern appropriation of the term concerns yet another polarity, that between passivity and activity.

And this is not at all a comprehensive overview of the matter. Quasi-contagious *pathos* is "the appeal of compassion triggered by the sight of suffering but also of awe in light of the self-possession on the part of those struck by misfortune", "the perseverance and dignity in the face of extreme calamity", and for the Christian passion (Christ's "passio"), it implies "a certain distance from and a way of overcoming pain in pain" (Buch, 2010, pp. 19–20). It "encompasses the tension between the appeal to a certain affective excess and the need to get this affective overload under control, precisely by casting it into a form, by fixating this intense vitality" (p. 21) (echoing Aby Warburg's (1999) *Pathosformel* or *pathos formula*; a fusion of a heightened affective state (Pathos) with a representational schema [Formel], an "engram of energy as expressive value" (p. 49)).

Maybe we need to stay a little longer on this specific notion of co-(m)-passion, co-suffering, the pathetic community (a community of *patheurs*) of the real world/cosmos, where every element is auto-affective, existing in and through this community, being intelligible to others and to oneself via the primal intelligibility of *pathos*, following Michel Henry's (2008, pp. 134–135) notion of *pathos-with*:

> Inasmuch as the essence of community is affectivity, the community is not limited to humans alone. It includes everything that is defined in itself by the primal suffering of life and thus by the possibility of suffering. We can suffer with everything that suffers. This pathos-with is the broadest form of every conceivable community.

But we need not forget that *pathos* as *pathos-with*, co(m)passion, co- or shared suffering, as a base for community and humanity and (maybe) as a new kind of universalism/humanism, the struggle against the "felt sense of precarity [...] that is at once singular and plural" (Butler, 2015, pp. 68–69), is just one of *pathos'* significances, the other one being (one might say) a "pathos of the real", "a sight all the more overwhelming for being beyond recognition and empathy", "a form of mourning that knows no consolation in the face of the destruction and suffering brought about by the failed encounters with the real" (Buch, 2010, p. 23).

Honig (2013, pp. 194–195), in her *Antigone, Interrupted*, wouldn't allow privileging public acts/performances over private communications/moves, wouldn't allow action to collapse into mourning, arguing that lamentation (no less than reason) "is itself an essentially contested and politicized practice", seeing/having stridency *together* with subtlety, pointing towards an *agonistic* humanism. Antigone's (speech) acts are not "comprehensively public" (Butler, 2000, p. 28), Honig (2013, p. 196) remarks, but *adianoeta*, paradoxical open secrets, a conspiratorial or covert form of communication, "a sort of pun or double entendre that carries 'two separate meanings, one "obvious" and one more subtle'", "various members of an audience will understand the same words differently" (p. 88).

Such is a glimpse to the breadth and depth (and height) of such a concept as *pathos*, its movements and changes, its demands and connotations and one would not want to enclose it, along with affect, emotion, feeling, etc. (and the relative network of other concepts, in close dialectical relationship), into just a narrow psychological concept.

Epopteia and *Elampsis*; *pathein*, being affected vs. *mathein*, being taught)

Pierre Boyancé (1962) tells us about one of the most important and transcendental senses of *pathos*. In his famous article, *Sur les mystères d' Éleusis*, he notes that there is substantial evidence of the effect produced by the mysteries, evidence which exposes very serious omissions on behalf of the significant work of Mylonas (1961), *Eleusis and the Eleusinian Mysteries*.

We shall present here just two small but crucial elements of Boyancé's treatise which tries to show that we are not in the dark regarding what constituted the rites of the *epopteia*: the viewing or "beholding, a kind of super-visionary seeing, a kind of essential panoptical vision, an *élampsis*, a direct, non-discursive illumination or contemplation". Even Plato in *Symposium* and *Phaedrus* appropriates the language of the Mysteries as a metaphor, an authoritative way of expressing his own (highest theoretical) vision, the kind of vision that real theory and philosophy is, the perfect knowledge, the contemplation of ideas, comparing them to an *epopteia* (Boyancé, 1962), something which, of course, echoes and reverberates not only to Neoplatonists but – if one dares to say it – even to the present day.

We find two important texts in Boyancé (1962, p. 462):

The first Aristotelean fragment could be translated as follows: "Those who have been perfected [the initiates] do not need to learn something, but rather undergo an experience and be brought into a certain state, having become, that is to say, fit [or receptive] for it." to learn something, but to be affected indicates two different modalities of knowing: *mathein* – intellectual learning through being taught/instructed, discursive learning, etc – and *pathein* – knowing by having experienced/suffered, by having been affected).

The second text could be translated as follows: "For all writing is divided into these two [kinds]: that which is God-breathed and the remaining part from the outside [education]; and [correspondingly] into the didactic and the *telestic* mode, i.e., pertaining to religious mysteries." The first, then, comes to men by hearing, but the second comes when the mind itself has undergone the illumination. This, indeed, is what Aristotle called mysterious and akin to the Eleusinian rites; for in those [rites] the initiate was being formed by the sacred visions but not being taught them. Instance of the mind itself undergoing illumination echoes the importance of this kind of excessive, experiential/experienced, passive illumination of *pathos*.

Clement of Alexandria (c. 150–c. 215 AD) was the Christian theologian and philosopher who rejected the idea of "the hyena's alternation of sexes", reiterating a "principle of the 'naturalness' of the male-female difference" (Foucault, 2021, p. 20), thus shaping the *aphrodisia* theme, or the right economy of pleasures, and a Christian way of relating to flesh. He notoriously attributed "the 'excessive' natural propensity for pleasure that characterizes the hyena" (p. 1) to a blameworthy, useless trait arguing about faith, truth, justice, and goodness, which can only be seen by the mind, not the eye:

A simple translation of the passage mentioned above could be this: "With good reason, then, the mysteries among the Greeks also begin with purifications, just as the bath does for the barbarians. After these are the Lesser Mysteries, which contain a certain foundation of instruction and of preparation for the things to come. The Greater Mysteries, however, are concerned with the universe as a whole, wherein nothing is left to be learned, but rather contemplated and comprehend both nature and things themselves." The verb *εποπτεύειν*, fused in the text, "surveying from above", means also "to behold", "to witness directly", paired up with another verb, *περινοεῖν*, "to" "apprehend", "grasp intellectually", "gain insight into", etc. A direct, revelatory, transformative vision *together with* a full, mental grasping of the nature of things and cosmos, for those who have seen, for the eyewitnesses (of the sacred visions).

Could a video camera capture from the outside the "inner vision of someone's mind-eye, someone who's having a deity-experience, an illumination induced either by an of old or new type of sacred, entheogenic drink like *kykeon*" (Wasson, Hofmann & Ruck, 1978) or through a transitory, liminal, psycho-somatic, mind-body-environment-sensory-diffused or unified *sense/sensing* (an overwhelming mind/eye-opening experience?

Maybe the true secret (the core) could not be betrayed; the experience (the *pathos*, the *affect*) was inexpressible, not articulable in words, even if the ritual acts (the shell) were described or even satirized; the experience could only be experienced.

Clement articulates (echoing and appropriating the Eleusinian marvel) a contrast, an antithesis, between (a lesser) and a greater learning: learning as discursive meaning-making and learning as a kind of "finding ourselves *into* sense/sensing a highly and deeply passive-affective transition, liminality and metamorphosis" (Boyancé, 1962, p. 462).

Actualized forms and forms in process of actualization

Stenner (2017) highlights a five-fold danger at play in the turn from discourse to affect with an analogy to a five-fold inspiration (p. 203). He notes that, after the structuralist "textual/discursive turn" (often referred to as "linguistic or cultural turn"), the "turn to affect" in the humanities continues and intensifies the project implicit in the discursive turn – the rejection of positivism – by rejecting the "onto-epistemological primacy of discourse" and giving centre stage to "whatever is not discourse" (p. 207). The implicit nature/culture bifurcation in the textual-turn methodology "privileges, when crudely handled, the cultural side of the distinction whilst leaving nature *as such* forever unspeakable" (p. 206), "by way of an insistence that nature is only knowable to us insofar as it is socially constructed as a part of our [...] culture" (p. 206). Consequently,

> unlike discourse, affect is not something we can collect, transcribe and analyse, and that is the point. It does not take an objective or public form that gives us the impression that we have it in front of us, like readable words on a page or recordable sounds in the air. Whatever affect is, it is not an "it" that can be designated by a "this". Whatever *this* is, it is not affect, since affect has already moved on and changed form. The affective turn stands up for this gesture of escape, and – in the name of affect – protects what escapes from being captured and frozen in discourse. [...] The affective turn stands up for those un-named and un-nameable possibilities that must forever remain virtual. Affect is not ... *yet*. Not *quite*.
>
> (Stenner, 2017, p. 208)

What *inspires* Stenner (2017) in a turn towards affect is *not exactly* such a notion of affect but the crucial point of the "processual contrast between actualized forms and forms in process of actualization", the "precarious emergence of novel forms" "on the edge of semantic availability", the liminal, transitory, lived, singular and vital "experience[s] of passage from one form to another", "enabled and enacted through the mediation of liminal affective technologies" (pp. 202–203).

What he also highlights, apart from the danger of daydreaming in the midst of serious catastrophic social and ecological events, is the danger of isolating "affect" as a "pristine state of primitive unqualified autonomy", harshly separating it from discourse or emotion, separating in this way what is fixed/explicit from what is vivid/living and implicit (following Gendlin's term, e.g., 1999, 2009), making it *merely* virtual, merely deconstructive and asubjective (p. 203).

The same crucial point as above, writes Stenner (2017), can be traced also in Spinoza's ontological distinction between the self-creating "Naturing nature" (*Natura naturans*) and all the creatures/creations that constitute "Natured nature" (*Natura naturata*), which applies to all forms of process, as well as in Alfred Schütz's (1945, p. 537) distinction between an ongoing process of acting in the living present (*actio*) and something done (in the past), performed, actualized (and reflected back upon) act (*actum*) and, finally, in Williams' (1977) distinction between forming/formative processes (of feeling/experience) and formed wholes (or units).

Auto-affection of life: *pathos* (affect) and *praxis* (force)

According to Davidson (2025), the maximalist phenomenology of life of Michel Henry (searching for the foundation of experience) and the minimalistic, humble, mediatory and conciliatory tone of Paul Ricoeur, and their dialogue, highlight anew the naturing/natured tension of nature and life and bring forth valuable new meaning regarding affectivity (p. 1). The lived experience of our own life, of our own living "original flesh" (p. 3), should be "the starting point and focus of any inquiry into life" (p. 2); this firsthand, subjective, feeling, which Henry calls the auto-affection/affectivity of life (p. 3), an original, pragmatic contact which needs to be restored (p. 4), the true immanent reality of life forgotten and concealed (p. 10). According to Henry, life is phenomenological because it is creative of phenomenality (p. 10). But what about the physical body and physiology? Is it "possible to speak about flesh without a body?" (p. 4). Ricoeur's hermeneutic phenomenology tries to reconcile "both the pragmatic and physiological perspectives toward the human" (p. 5).

This tension about ontological dependencies regarding the "pathos of life" and the quest for the most foundational origins of life and experience (the auto-manifestation of life vs. the manifestation of mundane things and the world) (pp. 182–183) highlights "the mutual interaction between one's own life and the lifeworld, between immanence and transcendence, between affect and representation, and, most importantly, between pathos and praxis"; the dialectic between the pathos of having a life and the praxis for leading a life, linking the subjective/internal experience of desire to the external circumstances and factors (biological, social, cultural, etc.) that shape it. Auto-affection of life, in a single expression, reveals the duality of the *pathos* (affect) (as an objective genitive) and the *praxis* (force, power to act) (as a subjective genitive) of life (p. 168) – *ordo essendi* and *ordo cognoscendi* forming a *living cogito* (p. 169) – both internal and external differences for both *pathos* and *praxis* – no sharp dichotomy between inner life and external world. The gift of life as a given and as a giving.

Affect in psychotherapy and education

Colette Soler (2016), trying to highlight what makes Lacanian psychoanalysis different from the varied forms of psychotherapy, writes:

> Psychoanalysis fosters the exploration of the unconscious, an unconscious that the subject does not know but that generates symptoms that affect him and that must be interpreted. Psychotherapy, on the contrary, welcomes the narration of affects that are not unconscious, that bother and preoccupy the patient, beginning with those that give rise to the various traumas that befall him in our world today.
>
> (p. 10)

For Soler, the Kierkegaardian affect of anguish (anxiety) can reveal "what the signifier cannot reveal: something real" (Soler, 2016, p. 21), something excluding meaning, something silent, "antinomical to all verisimilitude" (Lacan, 2001, p. 571). Anxiety possesses the "function" of a "true handle on reality" (an affective handle, not a symbolic Hegelian one): "the sole and final apprehension of any and all reality" derives "from that given to us by anguish" (Lacan, 2004, p. 385).

I am not sure if one "must choose between the two" (Lacan, 2004, p. 385), but I am sure that we need to distinguish concept(s) from affect(s), and not only regarding anguish, we need to acknowledge the interaction between meaning-making and the feeling process. Especially in those liminal phases and times when we, the speaking beings, are left adrift by the symbolic and the conceptual structures "to such an extent that" we "have been able to wonder if life is not a dream" (Soler, 2016, p. 20), when searching for our living vitality, our courage to live and die, for "the portion of life that is lost because of language" (p. 22) or even because of subjective or egoistic "truths".

Well, we are left adrift not just by the symbolic, but by life and death, and any kind of human and inhuman sufferings (we know that, for sure), having taken for some years our share of pleasures and pains, and, what is more, one needs not to adopt such a "structural" (Lacanian) view of antithesis or contradiction between different forms of therapy, exactly when (or due to the fact that) they have experienced the "truth" of anguish or even the "deceiving" immediate "non-truth" of other excessive, "enigmatic" affects. Anguish, *pathos*, excessive affects, delirium, the "failure to enjoy" as well as the "enjoyed knowledge" (Soler, 2016, p. 160), and the excessive actual somatic vibration of affective responsivity – the pathic dimension – go beyond our intentionality, understanding, causal logic, emerging "from the mysterious and impenetrable dimension from which experience originates" (Francesetti & Griffero, 2019, p. 41) and being situated "at the root of the emerging of the subject, when the subject has yet to be formed" (p. 41). By referring to the real, *pathos* (affect) – the opposite of apathy – can go beyond "the reach of the practice of speech and language" (p. 162). Patients suffer from what they feel, which implies that they are "not free to feel anything else. In this way, therapy [...] can be considered a process that broadens the freedom in responding to pathos in the therapy session" (p. 41).

Aristotle, defining *pathos* in a short sentence, writes in *De Anima:* "it is clear that the affections [of soul] are enfleshed accounts" (*De Anima*; C. D. C. Reeve, Trans., 2017), "enfleshed formulae", "formulable essences" etc. *Pathos* as *logos* enfleshed – something that reminds us of Lacan's human specificity as *parlêtre* – helps us to depart from the epistemology of translating *pathos* into *logos* and away from practices of, merely cognitive knowledge and manualized therapy, away from the logic of recognition *qua* category-identification/diagnosis; it is the enmattered or enfleshed *formation* or *Bildung*, and the personal encounter/contact/engagement, the embodying of attitudes and methods, that matter (Stanghellini in Francesetti & Griffero, 2019, pp. vii–viii). "There is a kind of knowledge that cannot simply be taught – it *must be learned*" (p. ix); it must be affecting/affected upon us, students, learners, therapy clients and therapists.

Taking the valuable (affective) *risk* of any kind of learning (either as students or clients, or just as living/dying beings) and navigating the flow and circulations of intensities of affects and affective processes are not about "to warn or not to warn", but, rather, about the question, "what is needed to take the risk in a given context?" (Kouri-Towe, 2023, p. 196).

An epilogue: desire and the *hyper*

Claire Colebrook (2023) sees "the significance of the anti-Oedipal work of Deleuze and Guattari [...] through a reconfiguration of gender and affect" (p. 9), locating gender-binaries and other "stabilities" (bodies with organs, social organization of bodies and flows, relations, etc.)

> within a broader history of desire, where desire is pre-human and pre-organic. Desire precedes, exceeds and disturbs the stabilities it brings into being, and might be thought of as radically affective. Affect is not something that happens to a body; it is through affective encounters that bodies come into being.
>
> (p. 10)

Desire "possesses more difference" (p. 9) than these stabilities: more complex, multiple differences, dynamic, inhuman/nonhuman. One needs even to do away with "an otherwise undifferentiated or asocial biology, life or matter" (p. 10). Affect and life are engendering and engendered. "Life comes into being from the relation among different forces – or forces to differ – that in turn enable recognizable differences. [...] [M]ore complex differences are reduced, diminished, flattened and rendered into stable forms" (p. 10).

I do not know if "*only* desire can explain the formations that emerge" (p. 10) in this anti-repressive, but productive model (of desire), or, in other words, I know that "desire" itself is just one of such formations.

We began this chapter by chasing *atmos*, vapour and *sphéra*, sphere: Schmitz's atmospheres, feelings, affects and affective powers as *quasi*-things, semantically ambiguous, vague, radically externalized, desubjectivized, situational, poured out like Homeric demons and felt-bodily qualities (both for the perceived forms and the perceivers), spatial but non-localizable, the "how" *qualia* of reality, rather than the "what" as defined/quantified materiality, the "pathic" rather than the "gnostic" (Francesetti & Griffero, 2019, pp. 1–3). We tried to present a kind of overview, to give a glimpse of a vast, vibrating, network of interwoven meanings about affect, pathos, mystery, life and death, pointing towards (actually) what it means to live (and die) better.

We don't need to fully follow this neo-phenomenological (affective) externalism. We might like to feel instead Gernot Böhme's (2017) humanistic *atmos+sphere* and his/its aesthetics (pp. 2–3). Not only for the "aesthetic professions" (psychotherapy included) but for everything and everyone who is not "'medusized' by an exclusively thingy orientation and by strictly functional parameters", expanding temporal to spatial, meaning-narration-representation to felt-bodily environmental-affective experience, positivist-statistical-quantifying predictions to phenomenic-atmospheric-feeling nuances, controlling-oppressing-repressing to the *pathic-affective* "more" (pp. 2–3).

Crudely, disciplinary power captures "affect" in "discourse", "by stabilizing collective liminal personae by ways of regimentation within institutional enclosures", with orders discursively organized, while the power of control (like in late capitalist aesthetic/affective economy) "continually modulates and stimulates the affect of 'dividuals' [...] suspending those controlled into a perpetual metastability of liminal potentiality" (Stenner, 2017, p. 210).

Maybe soon AI, like another Clement of Alexandria, will produce a similar text of appropriation, such as this chapter, drawing from fragments and representations (of affective procedure) and traces (of feelings) of the bright light, the bright darkness of hyper-death, hyper-life and hyper-reality (excuse me for this cryptic, this *αδιανόητο*, this open-secret).

So, unlike Clement or AI-the-transcriber-and-metonymizer, I want to announce and claim assured of my "personal identity through these absolute 'subjective facts'" (Francesetti & Griffero, 2019, p. 2) in such a "dead" and "dry" medium, the vitality *pathos* of affectivity, the *pathos* of receiving the gift of life, and the *secret*, or the *enigma*, the pain, the fear, the terror, the pleasure, the *aphrodisia*, the ecstasy, the heaven and the hell of what it means to live and die, a life-no-life and death-no-death, "excessively", like hyenas and hares, like human beings, "us", felt-living-bodies (*Leibs*), flesh and corpses, with love and care and compassion for any living creature, for the full power of (nuclear, infernal, reality-affective) bio-energy.

References

Αριστοτέλης. (1954). *Περί ψυχής – Μικρά Φυσικά* (Β. Τατάκης, Ν. Σωτηράκης, & Α. Ευσταθίου, Μεταφρ.· Ε. Π. Παπανούτσος, Επιμ.). Ι. Ζαχαρόπουλος. (Βιβλιοθήκη Αρχαίων Συγγραφέων, 15, 24). (Αρχικό έργο δημοσιευμένο περ. 350 π.Χ.).

Aristotle, (2017). *De Anima* (C. D. C. Reeve, Trans.). Hackett Publishing Company, Inc. (Original work published ca. 350 B.C.E.)

Auerbach, E. (1941). Passio als Leidenschaft. *Publications of the Modern Language Association of America*, *56*(4), 1179–1196.

Besnier, B., Moreau, P.- F., & Renault, L. (Eds.). (2003). *Les passions antiques et médiévales: Théories et critiques des passions, I*. Presses Universitaires de France.

Böhme, G. (2017). *The Aesthetics of Atmospheres*. Routledge.

Boyancé, P. (1962). Sur les mystères d'Éleusis. *Revue des Études Grecques*, *75*(356/358), 460–82.

Buch, R. (2010). *The Pathos of the Real. On the Aesthetics of Violence in the Twentieth Century*. The Johns Hopkins University Press.

Butler, J. (2000). *Antigone's Claim: Kinship between Life and Death*. Columbia University Press.

Butler, J. (2015). *Notes Toward a Performative Theory of Assembly*. Harvard University Press.

Colebrook, C. (2023). The Intense Germinal Influx. Affect as Engendering in Deleuze and Guattari. In Todd W. Reeser (Ed.), *The Routledge Companion to Gender and Affect* (pp. 9–22). Routledge.

Davidson, S. (2025). *Pathos and Praxis. An Integrated Phenomenology of Life*. Indiana University Press.

Dixon, T. (2003). *From Passions to Emotions. The Creation of a Secular Psychological Category*. Cambridge University Press.

Elsky, M. (2001). Introduction to Erich Auerbach, "Passio as Passion" ("Passio als Leidenschaft"). *Criticism, 43*(3), 285–308.

Francesetti, G. (2019). A Clinical Exploration of Atmospheres: Towards a Field-Based Clinical Practice. In G. Francesetti & T. Griffero (Eds.), *Psychopathology and Atmospheres: Neither Inside nor Outside*. Cambridge Scholars Publishing.

Francesetti, G., & Griffero, T. (Eds.). (2019). *Psychopathology and Atmospheres: Neither Inside nor Outside*. Cambridge Scholars Publishing. pp 2–50.

Foucault, M. (2021). *Confessions of the Flesh: The History of Sexuality, Volume 4*. Knopf Doubleday Publishing Group.

Fuchs, T. (1995). Coenästhesie. Zur Geschichte des Gemeingefühls. *Z Klin Psychol Psychother, 43*, 103–112.

Fuchs, T. (2018). *Ecology of the Brain: The Phenomenology and Biology of the Embodied Mind*. Oxford University Press.

Gendlin, E. T. (1996). *Focusing-Oriented Psychotherapy*. Guilford.

Gendlin, E. T. (1999). Implicit entry and focusing. *The Humanistic Psychologist, 27*, 1, 80–88. From https://www.focusing.org/gendlin/docs/gol_2032.html

Gendlin, E. T. (2009). We Can Think with the Implicit, as Well as with Fully Formed Concepts. In Karl Leidlmair (Ed.), *After Cognitivism: A Reassessment of Cognitive Science and Philosophy* (pp. 147–161). Springer.

Green, A. (1977). The Conception of Affect. *International Journal of Psychoanalysis, 58*(2), 129–56.

Griffero, T. (2024). *Being a Lived Body*. Routledge.

Harris, W. V. (2001). *Restraining Rage: The Ideology of Anger Control in Classical Antiquity*. Harvard University Press.

Hearn, J. (2021). Serious Emotions: On Some Emotions in Working on Men's Violences and Violences to Women. In M. Husso, S. Karkulehto, T. Saresma, A. Laitila, J. Eilola, & H. Siltala (Eds.), *Violence, Gender and Affect. Interpersonal, Institutional and Ideological Practices*. Palgrave Macmillan, pp. 80–93.

Henry, M. (2008). *Material Phenomenology* (S. Davidson, Trans.). Fordham University Press.

Konstan, D. (2006). *The Emotions of the Ancient Greeks: Studies in Aristotle and Classical Literature*. University of Toronto Press.

Kouri-Towe, N. (2023). Affective Pedagogies, and Pedagogies of Affect. Gender, Solidarity, and the Classroom in the Trigger Warning Debates. In T. W. Reeser (Ed.), *The Routledge Companion to Gender and Affect* (pp. 188–198). Routledge.

Lacan, J. (2001). *Autres écrits* (Other writings) (J.- A. Miller, Ed.). Seuil.

Lacan, J. (2004). *Le séminaire de Jacques Lacan, Livre X: L'angoisse (1962–1963)* (The seminar of Jacques Lacan, book X: Anxiety.) (J.-A. Miller, Ed.). Seuil.

Langer, S. (1953). *Feeling and Form*. Routledge.

Leikert, S. (2019). *Das sinnliche Selbst: Körpergedächtnis und psychoanalytische Behandlungstechnik*. Brandes & Apsel.
Massumi, B. (1995). The Autonomy of Affect. *Cultural Critique*, *31*(2), 83–109.
Massumi, B. (2002). *Parables for the Virtual: Movement, Affect, Sensation*. Duke University Press.
Moreau, P.-F. (2003). Τα πάθη [στην κλασική εποχή]: Γενική προβληματική (Γ. Πρελορέντζος, Μεταφρ.). *Δωδώνη: Μέρος Τρίτο, Επιστημονική Επετηρίδα του Τμήματος Φιλοσοφίας, Παιδαγωγικής και Ψυχολογίας*, *32*, 33–48.
Moreau, P.- F., & Ramond, C. (Eds.). (2006). *Les passions à l'âge classique: Théories et critiques des passions, II*. Presses Universitaires de France.
Mylonas, G. E. (1961). *Eleusis and the Eleusinian Mysteries*. Princeton University Press.
Oele, M. (2020). *E-Co-Affectivity. Exploring Pathos at Life's Material Interfaces*. Sunny Press.
Reeser, T. W. (2023). The Affect of Gender, the Gender of Affect. In T. W. Reeser (Ed.), *The Routledge Companion to Gender and Affect* (pp. 3–8). Routledge.
Richards, G., & Stenner, P. (2023). *Putting Psychology in Its Place. Critical Historical Perspectives* (4th ed.). Routledge.
Scapin, N. (2020). *The Flower of Suffering. Theology, Justice, and the Cosmos in Aeschylus' Oresteia and Presocratic Thought*. De Gruyter.
Schmitz, H. (2019). *New Phenomenology. A Brief Introduction* (T. Griffero, Ed.). Mimesis International.
Schmitz, H. (2023). *Atmospheres*. Mimesis International.
Schultz-Venrath, U. (2024). *Mentalizing the Body. Integrating Body and Mind in Psychotherapy*. Routledge.
Schütz, A. (1945). On Multiple Realities. *Philosophy and Phenomenological Research*, *5*(4), 533–76.
Sedgwick, E. K., & Frank, A. (1995). Shame in the Cybernetic Fold: Reading Silvan Tomkins. *Critical Inquiry*, *21*(2), 496–505.
Soler, C. (2016). *Lacanian Affects. The Function of Affect in Lacan's Work* (B. Fink, Trans.). Routledge.
Sommerstein, A. H. (2010). *Aeschylean Tragedy*. Bloomsbury.
Spinoza, B. ([1677] 1989). *Ethics: Including the Improvement of the Understanding* (R. H. M. Elwes, Trans.). Prometheus books.
Stenner, P. (2017). *Liminality and Experience: A Transdisciplinary Approach to the Psychosocial*. Palgrave Macmillan.
Stern, D. N. (2010). *Forms of Vitality. Exploring Dynamic Experience in Psychology, the Arts, Psychotherapy, and Development*. Oxford University Press.
Szakolczai, Á. (2009). Liminality and Experience: Structuring Transitory Situations and Transformative Events. *International Political Anthropology*, *2*(1), 141–72.
Szakolczai, Á. (2016). *Permanent Liminality and Modernity*. Routledge.
Tomkins, S. (1962). *Affect, Imagery, Consciousness* (Vol. 1). Springer Publishing Company.
Turner, V. (1969/1995). *The Ritual Process: Structure and Anti-Structure*. Aldine de Gruyter.
Turner, V. (1982). *From Ritual to Theatre: The Human Seriousness of Play*. PAJ.
Van Gennep, A. (1909/1961). *The Rites of Passage*. University of Chicago Press.
Warburg, A. (1999). *The Renewal of Pagan Antiquity: Contributions to the Cultural History of the European Renaissance* (D. Britt, Trans.). Getty Research Institute for the History of Art and the Humanities. (Original work published 1932).

Wasson, R. G., Hofmann, A., & Ruck, C. A. P. (1978). *The Road to Eleusis*. Harcourt Brace Jovanovich.
Wetherell, M. (2012). *Affect and Emotion: A New Social science Understanding*. Sage.
Wetherell, M. (2013). Affect and Discourse – What's the Problem? From Affect as Excess to Affective/Discursive Practice. *Subjectivity*, *6*(4), 349–368.
Whitehead, A. N. (1929/1985). *Process and Reality*. The Free Press.
Williams, R. (1977). *Marxism and Literature*. Oxford University Press.

Chapter 14

Encounter in everyday life as affective dialogue

Bridging the individual and the collective

Agniya Pasechnik-Lyle

Introduction

This chapter revisits the concept of *encounter* through the lens of affect theory and everyday life. While *encounter* has long been central to humanistic psychology (Bugental, 1965; Gendlin, 1981; May, 1969; Rogers, 1961; Yalom, 1980), especially in the therapeutic context, this work aims to extend its scope by tracing how resonance and transformation arise in ordinary relational moments. Building on grounded theory research (Pasechnik-Lyle & Kharkhurin, 2024), and drawing from the psychological framework rooted in Rogers (1970) to philosophical perspectives such as Spinoza's (1996), it explores how *affect* moves us into relation, how the self comes forward through resonance, and how certain *encounters* leave affective traces that shape not only the individual but the emotional climate of the collective. This chapter unfolds in three movements: from affective dialogue and resonance to a structural *continuum of encounter*, and finally to the notion of *resonant encounter* as a living field—a shared affective space that remembers, reshapes, and connects.

Encounter as affective dialogue

In the humanistic tradition, *encounter* refers to a moment of genuine presence between individuals—a relational space where congruence, empathy, and unconditional regard can catalyse personal transformation (Rogers, 1970). While classically situated in therapeutic contexts, this concept can be extended to the ordinary spaces of life, where meaningful contact emerges in conversations, gestures, and silences, wherever two people meet in realness.

Here we take *encounter* out of the clinical frame and into the relational texture of daily life. What happens in those moments when something in us is stirred by another? When do we feel not only seen, but sensed? At the core of these moments lies *affect*—the pre-personal, embodied intensity that moves between bodies before language has shaped it (Bazzano, 2020).

As Spinoza (1996) articulated, affect is the body's power to affect and be affected. It is not emotion in the psychological sense, but the underlying dynamic that gives rise to emotion and feeling. Following Massumi (1995), affect is immediate and

DOI: 10.4324/9781003669906-15

relational—a force that registers before it is understood, forming the atmospheric ground of experience. It shapes our openness, our defences, our readiness to connect or withdraw.

In encounter, affect moves from an internal sensation to a relational phenomenon. It does not stay sealed within a single subject. It reaches outward, seeking contact, seeking reflection. This subtle interplay of bodily presence, tone, and timing is what we refer to as affective dialogue: a process through which affect becomes relationally meaningful, even before it becomes linguistically clear. Such attunement has been described by Schore (2001) as a right-brain-to-right-brain synchronization that underpins affective resonance in early development and beyond.

Rather than focusing solely on cognitive understanding or verbal communication, this perspective emphasizes how transformation emerges through the feeling field that unfolds between people. Meaningful encounter occurs not only when we are understood, but when we are *felt into being*. And this felt recognition, even when brief, can reshape the awareness in relation to others. In this way, affect is not simply an inner sensation, but a bridge between self and other.

From affect to feeling: the invisible movements of encounter

At the heart of every encounter lies affect—a force of intensity, a bodily readiness to feel, connect, and respond (Spinoza, 1996). It is not an emotion, not yet a feeling, but a surge, a shift, a trembling. It moves through us often without form, setting the tone of an interaction before we consciously know what we are responding to (Massumi, 1995).

This intensity, however, does not stay shapeless. As it interacts with another body, with a gaze, a silence, a gesture—it begins to take on sense. Sense is the first contouring of affect. It does not offer clarity, but it gives direction. We may suddenly feel drawn toward someone, or slightly guarded, without knowing why (Damasio, 1999). Something is happening, and we register it with our whole being. Sense is how affect begins to speak.

As that speaking becomes clearer, feeling emerges. Gendlin (1981) described this as the felt sense—the body's way of knowing more than the mind can say. Feelings offer us a bridge: between what stirs inside and what we can begin to understand, between what is ours and what is shared. In encounter, they shape the quality of the relational field: its warmth, its charge, its openness, or resistance. Feelings are personal and then expressed in emotions that are reflections of feelings in social settings (Massumi, 1995).

Affect, sense, feeling, and emotion are not stages in a linear sequence. They are overlapping movements in the choreography of connection. Sometimes, feeling arrives swiftly and clearly. Other times, we dwell in the ambiguity of sense. But always, affect is there, setting the pulse beneath the interaction.

Even before a word is spoken, two people in proximity are already engaging in an unspoken negotiation of presence. Their bodies are reading one another, attuning, deciding whether to open or close. As Fuchs (2016) suggests, affect is what moves through the space between us—it shapes the very possibility of encounter, he articulates: it is "intuitive understanding of others' emotions in our embodied engagement with them" (Fuchs, 2016, p. 4).

Before empathy, before intention, before dialogue, there is this subtle charge that says: something real might happen here.

In this way, affect is not just what we feel. It is what makes feeling and relation possible. But not all affective intensities are alike. While affect is neutral in origin, a pre-personal stirring, a bodily potential, it becomes charged through experience. Memory, attention, early relational patterns, and even unspoken cultural scripts begin to colour the field. Affective states take shape as echoes of what has been felt before, or what the body anticipates might be felt again. This is why, in certain moments, a simple glance, silence, or gesture can carry a disproportionate emotional weight: the field is not empty, but already resonant with prior affective life.

Affective resonance: the bridge that feels us into being

If affect is the silent current beneath all interaction, *resonance* is the moment that current becomes relational. Massumi (1995) writes: "the level of intensity and qualification is not one of conformity or correspondence, but of resonance" (Massumi, 1995, p. 86). Rosa (2019) describes resonance as a felt response, a moment of deep attunement where one's inner world is acknowledged and amplified by another. *Affective resonance* occurs when two individuals attune to each other's affective states, amplifying and shaping the emotional energy of an interaction. This process bridges the gap between internal experience and relational meaning, turning raw affect into a shared, embodied experience (Fuchs, 2016). Resonance does not occur simply because one person feels. It arises when that feeling is met, sensed, received, and echoed through the presence of another. In such moments, affect moves through interiority to shared space. It becomes felt between, not only within. The body responds, the atmosphere thickens, and something unspeakable is quietly named.

Feeling becomes the language that resonance speaks, not in the form of interpretation or analysis, but as a tuning between beings. The field itself begins to vibrate differently. What begins as a subtle sensation can swell into clarity or even transformation (Bazzano & Webb, 2016). Dissanayake (2000) describes similar bioaffective mirroring in early mother-infant interactions, arguing that such rhythmic, emotionally charged exchanges are the roots not only of empathy but of art itself. In this light, resonance may be seen as a deeply patterned human capacity to co-regulate, co-create, and create meaning through embodied affective attunement.

As resonance deepens, emotion takes shape, sometimes gentle, sometimes raw. Yet all such feelings carry the potential to reconfigure the inner landscape. Affective resonance does not merely affirm what we already know—it *reshapes* us. In the right conditions, emotion moves from latency into expression, from ambiguity into form. We are altered not through explanation, but through being felt into being.

Longing as the voice of affect

Often, what surfaces in moments of resonance is not just a definable feeling, but a *longing*—a wish that stretches beyond the awareness. Longing is the voice of affect calling out for meaningful presence. It signals that the space between awareness and the other has become charged with possibility. In Lacanian theory, desire arises precisely where presence is elusive, as a structuring absence that animates the subject (Lacan, 1998).

Across both therapeutic sessions and ordinary encounters, I've observed how this longing appears—tentative, truthful, and deeply affective. A client recently shared, "I want to truly feel needed." A stranger on a long train ride, in the kind of moment where masks soften, said almost the same words. These weren't confessions in the usual sense. They were declarations of resonance—a desire not for romance or approval, but for communion. For the space between two people to matter so deeply that, without the other, it could not fully exist.

Someone names a need directly or obliquely, not just to be answered, but to be met. What they carry inside seeks not advice, but a felt resolution. They long to be seen not as a problem to solve, but as a being whose vulnerability matters. They want what is in between to be real, to change them both. Often, those who voice such longings do so because they intuit something in you: a capacity to hear what hasn't yet been said. A way of holding what trembles, without rushing to interpret or fix. To meet longing with presence is to participate in its unfolding. And perhaps, to be changed by it as well.

The encounter that changes us

Ultimately, resonance is not about comfort. It is about truth. Cognitive awareness alone does not transform. Transformation occurs in the moment when emotion is not only allowed but also received, reflected, and gently named. When two beings meet not merely through speech but through attuned feeling, something shifts. Encounter becomes more than interaction—it becomes a movement of emotional truth, where affect finds form through relation.

Not all resonance soothes. Some disturb. Some confront. Some stir what had remained unvoiced, the silent intensities at the edges of self-experience. Yet these moments are not deviations; they are proof of contact. Discomfort, then, may signal not wounding, but the threshold of becoming, a moment where something within us is being exposed as potential. This is often what holds people back from entering the encounter: not fear of the other, but uncertainty about their readiness to feel what awareness is about to expose. Yet every new moment carries a new feeling, and if it is received, it becomes an invitation to become. In this sense, affect is not just the content of feeling; it is the vector of becoming.

In my recent research, such moments were often described as transformative (Pasechnik-Lyle, 2025). They left an imprint, a residue that lingered in the body and atmosphere. And across those accounts, a shared rhythm began to emerge, a vibration of unfolding. What follows is a synthesis of those insights—a conceptual arc of how affective resonance tends to move:

- Affective awakening—the first stirrings of aliveness, often ambiguous or pre-verbal. These resemble what Deleuze (1990) calls "affects without subjects"—emergent forces that have not yet entered the register of identity or emotion.
- Affective recognition—the moment when feeling begins to cohere, intuitively grasped, or softly named. This is not yet interpretation, but what Fuchs (2016) called embodied interaffectivity, where relational presence helps pre-reflective affect become felt as one's own.
- Affective integration—when emotion becomes meaning, not through analysis, but through embodied belonging. Here, awareness unfolds as resonant synthesis, a convergence of body, feeling, and relation into affective sense.

This arc does not prescribe how every encounter should move, but shows how, when resonance is allowed to do its work, we often find ourselves moved from numbness to sensation, from solitude to relation, from fragmentation to coherence. In this way, resonance becomes the bridge that feels us into being, an event of becoming-with.

While affect may begin as an internal stirring and resonance may draw us toward the other, what happens next, how we meet, unfold, and transform, follows a rhythm. To explore this rhythm is to trace what Deleuze and Guattari (1987) call a "line of flight"—the subtle path by which new forms of subjectivity emerge.

Analysis of the encounter narratives (Pasechnik-Lyle & Khakhurin, 2024) revealed that the most significant variable shaping the experience was the individual's mode of perceiving. Some people shared that they never had an experience of encounter; others described it as rare but valuable; still others lived as though encounter were a daily orientation, a way of life. Tellingly, all acknowledged such moments as existentially meaningful, but not all were willing to engage. The natural question follows: If it is so meaningful, why does one hold back? Those who had never experienced an encounter often expressed the belief that such moments are impossible: people wear masks, people lie, people always want something. "I wish I could believe in it," one participant said, "but I just don't think it's real." This cognitive rigidity seems to confine the awareness, preventing it from approaching what is most longed for. We called this mode the *organismic* (Rogers, 1959), a felt sense that encounter exists, paired with a refusal to enter it.

Others recognized encounters as rare but possible. These participants seemed reflective, connected to their emotions, and what Fusch (2016) describes as *affective affordances*. They described moments when something opened up inside them, even if briefly. That moment of affective recognition settled into awareness. Their descriptions aligned with what Gendlin (1981) calls the felt sense: experience deeply sensed and allowed to unfold. We named this mode of perceiving as *bodily*.

Still others described encounter as essential to life. They actively sought it, even in mundane interactions. Those people were reflective not only about its presence, but also about its meaning and consequences. This mode of perceiving we named the *mindful*, where awareness is engaged in the ongoing process of living life in relation. These modes of perceiving reflect how affect is sensed, metabolized, and transformed into meaning. One might say that at the core of the experience of encounter lies a fundamental faith in its possibility, its reality, and its existential significance.

If careful following of deep connection teaches us anything, it's that understanding rarely follows a straight line. We do not move cleanly from beginning to end. Instead, we circle, spiral, pause, and return, again and again, to parts of ourselves once thought is resolved. So, what became apparent was that the experience of encounter breathes—it follows a cycling pattern. We observed two recurring movements in participants' narratives. These are not linear stages, but rhythmic cycles that echo the natural respiration of relational life.

- The *Cycle of Discovery* begins when something within us awakens. It may be a rupture, a longing, or quiet discontent. Affect begins to stir. We become more porous, more curious. This resonance, though subtle, signals readiness.
- The *Cycle of Exploration* follows. Here, we lean into connection. We allow vulnerability. Resonance deepens. But progress is not guaranteed. We may stall or return to discovery. These cycles recur across the lifespan. After moments that support our awareness to expand and sense more, we are called back into quiet rediscovery. Often, solitude was mentioned as a necessary choice for integration, as if the body asks for space to metabolize what it has met.

As we move through encounters, something in our way of experiencing shifts. We begin with sensation, move to feeling, and arrive at insights that feel both intimate and vast. These are not fixed stages but modulations of affective intensity. They reflect where the flow of affect is smooth or where it stagnates, and why. Fuchs (2016) writes that the intercorporeal field remembers not through narrative, but through repetition and rhythm. We feel again what has been once felt, not as memory, but as potential returning. And so, what was once a private sensation becomes a shared affect. Connection becomes becoming.

Resonant encounter as an affective field: the space that remembers us

We explored encounter as an unfolding rhythm, from the stirrings of affect to the resonance that reshapes awareness. We followed the inner logic of how connection awakens, moves, deepens, and transforms. But some encounters do not end when the interaction ceases. Their affective charge remains, sometimes quietly, sometimes insistently, shaping us long after the moment has passed. What follows is not a departure from the previous inquiry, but an expansion: from encounter as an event to what I call a *resonant encounter*—an ongoing atmosphere of relation, memory, and becoming.

Carl Rogers (1970) originally conceived encounter as a transformative moment of authentic meeting between persons—a moment of truth and change. In honouring that origin, I extend the idea into a wider relational field, drawing on affect theory to suggest that encounters continue not just in memory, but in the body, in the emotional atmosphere, and in the ongoing becoming of the awareness.

Encounter as affective atmosphere: from event to field

Affect theorists describe affect not as a personal emotion, but as a dynamic field, a set of intensities that move across bodies, space, and time. Massumi (1995) emphasizes that affect is atmospheric and non-linear; it exceeds the boundaries of individual identity. Spinoza, much earlier, argued that affects are modes of existence, changes in the body's capacity to act, shaped by encounters with other bodies. Deleuze and Guattari (1987) extend this notion, conceptualizing affect as part of a 'plane of immanence,' where beings co-constitute each other through flows of force. In this view, relation precedes individuality: to affect and be affected is to become.

An encounter, then, is not merely an experience between two people. It is a relational field, a charged space that holds emotional intensity, impression, and potential. It is a process of *co-being*, where parties emerge through mutual transformation. Berlant (2011) describes such affective fields as "situations where something is felt before it can be said and endured before it is understood." To see this way is to shift perspective: from a moment to a continuum, from a single interaction to a field in motion, from isolated individuals to a shared energetic field that continues to live within and around us.

Integration through distance: solitude and becoming

There are times when we are alone yet feel someone else's presence within us. These are not memories alone, they are affective traces, remnants of a resonance that once shaped us and perhaps still does. In solitude, the body begins to reorganize what it once experienced in connection. A breath tightens. A thought reemerges. A new insight arises. These are not regressions, but phases of integration, essential moments in the rhythm of encounter.

Such integration is not an act of will. It happens subtly, like dusk becoming night. The awareness reshapes in response to what was felt. And in that reshaping, a new readiness may form for the next encounter, for a deeper presence, or for a quiet truth now ready to be lived.

Learning from the affective field

To conceptualize encounter as an affective field is to recognize that our connections are not isolated or accidental. They are part of a living, moving, intelligent web. Some people enter our lives not only to connect, but to reveal. To reflect something back that is ready to be seen (Pasechnik-Lyle & Kharkhurin, 2024). And some encounters arrive not to stay, but to open, like a window or a song.

The more we become attuned to the affective field, the more we recognize that our presence matters, that we are always shaping and being shaped. That we are not only touched by others, but carriers of resonance ourselves. This is when that longing to be needed gradually satisfies. It opens us to the possibility that each resonant encounter, even the smallest, may be part of a larger kaleidoscope of meaning.

Even when two people part, the resonance they created does not dissolve. It stays in the body, in memory, in atmosphere. It may return in dreams, in a piece of music, or a sudden wave of feeling. It may shape how we enter the next interaction or how we choose to be alone.

In this sense, an encounter is not something we "had," but something we entered and which continues to unfold within us. It becomes part of our emotional architecture. Once two people meet in resonance, a thread is spun between them, and that thread remembers.

The shifting nature of affect ensures that no encounter stays the same. What felt one way yesterday may feel entirely different tomorrow. The same experience may be re-lived, re-felt, and re-understood over time. This is why encounter is recursive, we revisit it, internally or relationally, sometimes long after the moment has passed. Berardi (2009) describes how affective labour and social interaction recursively shape not only individual states but also the collective emotional economy, pointing to the psychic toll of contemporary relational life and its potential for renewal. He writes that "we must see it as an anthropological turning point that is going to change the distribution of world resources and of world power" (Berardi, 2009, p. 212). In this light, affect is not only personal or relational, it is historical. Each thread of resonance participates in a larger weave, linking the intimate to the planetary.

When we understand encounter as a relational field, we no longer ask whether something "meant" enough. We begin instead to ask: What has it opened in me? What has it left alive? What thread continues to vibrate, quietly, through my life?

We are never untouched by those we have met in resonance. Even the briefest contact can alter the emotional terrain of awareness. Encounter is not something we can hold, but something we can feel moving through us. And perhaps, in becoming aware of that movement, we begin to live differently—more attuned, more spacious, more open.

Encounter and the collective: affective patterns beyond the individual

Over time, resonant threads extend beyond individual lives, forming affective patterns across relationships, communities, and cultures. When sustained, these patterns crystallize into a *cultural atmosphere*—a shared emotional climate that subtly guides how we feel, speak, and relate. This transformation from internal resonance to shared intensity reflects what Clough and Halley (2007) call the *affective turn*:

a shift beyond language and representation toward embodiment, circulation, and the social life of feeling. Affect, in this view, is not contained—it is transindividual (Simondon, 2020). It moves through us and between us, creating the unseen fabric of collective life. Bazzano (2025) captures this beautifully: "[the notion of] separate individuals is an attractive illusion and a second-rate mode of being in the world—a private that is deprived existence, depriving us of the rich transindividual nature of our individuality" (Bazzano, 2025, p. 143). Encounter undoes this illusion. It reveals that individuality emerges not in isolation, but through shared becoming.

To live attentively to encounter is, then, not only to meet another more fully—it is to help shape the emotional architecture of our shared world. This aligns with Barad's (2007) concept of *intra-action*, where matter and meaning emerge not from discrete subjects but from relational entanglement. Through this lens, encounter is not just an intimate moment, but a world-making process—one that is emotional, ethical, and material.

Conclusion: living the affective continuum

What began as a fleeting moment between bodies—a glance, a silence, a surge of feeling—has unfolded into a complex, dynamic field of meaning. This chapter traced how encounter, long cherished in humanistic psychology as a moment of authenticity, expands under the lens of affect theory into a rhythmic, ongoing process of becoming. We have moved from affect as a preverbal stirring, through resonance as the bridge of mutual recognition and emotional integration that expands awareness.

Along the way, we came to see that encounter is not limited to the therapy room, nor even to intimate moments. It is an ever-present possibility within the emotional texture of everyday life, waiting to be recognized, felt, and lived. Affect doesn't just pass between individuals; it leaves imprints, reshapes relational tendencies, and, when echoed across time and space, forms the affective fabric of our shared world.

The notion of resonant encounter emerges not as a reinvention of Rogers' vision, but as its unfolding. It offers a language for the recursive, embodied, and often ineffable nature of meaningful connection—one that continues to act upon us long after the initial contact. To meet another in affect is to invite some part of the awareness to come forward; to be met in return is to join in the slow work of shaping the relational field that holds us all.

This understanding bridges the personal and the collective. The transformation that begins in the terrain of the body extends outward, shaping relationships, group dynamics, and cultural atmospheres. When we attune to the affective field, we become not just more fully ourselves, but more ethically present in the world. This reconceptualization of encounter draws together Rogers' (1970) humanistic ideal of authentic meeting, Spinoza's (1996) insight into affective capacity, and Massumi's (1995) theory of embodied intensity, reweaving these into a model of relational becoming grounded in everyday life.

To live attuned to encounter, then, is a political and spiritual act. It is to resist fragmentation, to refuse numbness, and to step again and again into the risk and beauty of relation. Not every contact will change us, but any moment might. And each time we allow affect to move, each time we meet or are met in resonance, we affirm the truth at the heart of this chapter: we come into being together, or as Barad (2007) writes, we are not separate entities interacting, but entangled phenomena, "I" am a "We" (Spinoza, 1996).

References

Barad, K. (2007). *Meeting the universe halfway: Quantum physics and the entanglement of matter and meaning*. Durham, NC: Duke University Press.

Bazzano, M. (2020). *The Skin is faster than the Word*. Hermeneutic Circular. https://doi.org/10.4324/9781003280262-18

Bazzano, M., & Webb, J. (Eds.). (2016). *Therapy and the counter-tradition: The edge of philosophy*. London: Routledge.

Bazzano, M. (2025). On transindividuation. Or: How can we overcome the enduring split between individuals and society? *European Journal of Psychotherapy & Counselling*, 27(1–2), 138–151. https://doi.org/10.1080/13642537.2024.2403433

Benjamin, J. (1988). *The bonds of love: Psychoanalysis, feminism, and the problem of domination*. Pantheon Books.

Berardi, F. (2009). *The soul at work: From alienation to autonomy* (F. Cadel & G. Mecchia, Trans.). Semiotext(e). (Original work published 2007)

Berlant, L. (2011). *Cruel optimism*. Duke University Press.

Bugental, J. F. T. (1965). *The search for authenticity: An existential-analytic approach to psychotherapy*. Holt, Rinehart and Winston.

Clough, P. T., & Halley, J. (Eds.). (2007). *The affective turn: Theorizing the social*. Durham, NC: Duke University Press.

Damasio, A. R. (1999). *The feeling of what happens: Body and emotion in the making of consciousness*. New York: Harcourt Brace.

Deleuze, G., & Guattari, F. (1987). *A thousand plateaus: Capitalism and schizophrenia* (B. Massumi, Trans.). University of Minnesota Press. (Original work published 1980)

Deleuze, G. (1990). *The logic of sense* (M. Lester & C. Stivale, Trans. ; C. Boundas, Ed.). Columbia University Press. (Original work published 1969)

Dissanayake, E. (2000). *Art and intimacy: How the arts began*. University of Washington Press.

Fuchs, T. (2016). *Intercorporeality and interaffectivity. Phenomenology and the Cognitive Sciences*. Oxford University Press. 15(3), 413–31. https://doi.org/10.1007/s11097-015-9437-4

Gendlin, E. T. (1981). *Focusing*. New York: Bantam Books.

Lacan, J. (1998). *The four fundamental concepts of psychoanalysis* (J.- A. Miller, Ed., A. Sheridan, Trans.). New York: W. W. Norton. (Original work published 1973)

Massumi, B. (1995). The autonomy of affect. *Cultural Critique*, 31, 83–109. https://doi.org/10.2307/1354446

May, R. (1969). *Love and will*. New York: W.W. Norton & Company.

Pasechnik-Lyle, A. (2025). The dual work of Encounter: Shaping the self through intrapersonal and interpersonal experience. *Human Being: Image and Essence. Humanitarian Aspects*, 4.

Pasechnik-Lyle, A., & Kharkhurin, A. (2024). The architectures of encounter: A grounded theory study of authentic communication and self-discovery in everyday life. *Journal of Constructivist Psychology*. https://doi.org/10.1080/10720537.2024.2388037

Rogers, C. R. (1959). A theory of therapy, personality, and interpersonal relationships as developed in the client-centered framework. In S. Koch (Ed.), *Psychology: A study of a science*. Vol. 3: *Formulations of the person and the social context* (pp. 184–256). New York: McGraw-Hill.

Rogers, C. R. (1961). *On becoming a person: A therapist's view of psychotherapy*. Boston, MA: Houghton Mifflin.

Rogers, C. R. (1970). *Encounter groups*. New York: Harper & Row.

Rosa, H. (2019). *Resonance: A sociology of our relationship to the world* (J. C. Wagner, Trans.). Cambridge: Polity Press.

Schore, A. N. (2001). The effects of early relational trauma on right brain development, affect regulation, and infant mental health. *Infant Mental Health Journal*, 22(1–2), 201–269. https://doi.org/10.1002/1097-0355(200101/04)22:1<201::AID-IMHJ8>3.0.CO;2-9

Simondon, G. (2020). *Individuation in light of notions of form and information* (T Adkins, Trans.). Minneapolis, MN: University of Minnesota Press.

Spinoza, B. (1996). *Ethics* (E. Curley, Trans.). Princeton, NJ: Princeton University Press. (Original work published 1677)

Wilber, K. (1995). *Sex, ecology, spirituality: The spirit of evolution*. Boulder, CO: Shambhala.

Yalom, I. D. (1980). *Existential psychotherapy*. New York: Basic Books.

Chapter 15

Reality, but not as we know it

Seb Heid

"The owls are not what they seem"

It's quite a popular topic in popular culture that reality cannot be trusted. Not just since we entered the age of fake news and AI-generated content that can fool everybody. We are living in a Matrix. This colourful experience of mine might be nothing but the fever dream of a drunken demon.

The question "What is reality?" can easily mess with people's minds, which explains its ubiquitous presence in the subtext of thriller/horror/sci-fi movie plots, but also why philosophers and psychologists keep coming back to it. Despite a longstanding tradition to the contrary, people don't actually perceive the world as objective neutral facts. Of course, at least since Kant, there is a growing awareness that it would be wrong to assume that the world exists in the shape of neatly packaged facts just waiting for us to be perceived. The construction of reality is messy business, and while Kant might have still put a lot of hope in our ability to construct some rationally ordered world, it has become clear since then that making sense of our reality is not just a matter of rational analysis.

Therapy can be one way of helping people make sense of themselves and their reality. When it works, it can feel like magic, and it is always intriguing when something feels magical. Following the hunch by Arthur C. Clarke (1972) that any significantly advanced technology is indistinguishable from magic, the sense of something feeling like magic is an irresistible invitation to try to understand the complex inner workings of the "thing" in question. What does that mean for therapy? What is the connection between therapy and making sense of our reality? How does therapy work? Exploring potential answers to these questions brings up more questions, for instance: What does it mean to make sense of something? What does it mean to have a reality? How can therapy assist that process? As a guide to this thicket of questions, I want to suggest a model of therapy that centres on one core idea: *affect*.

Often ignored, affect is the key ingredient of the reality that we need to understand. Affect is what creates the connection between therapist and client. By finding ways of making sense of affect, the conditions are created that allow the client to make progress in their endeavour of understanding their unique reality and of who they are within that reality.

DOI: 10.4324/9781003669906-16

Most importantly, affect connects with the visceral sense that the whole world isn't quite what it seems.

A sense of what is missing – Why reality is far too important to leave it to the logicians or linguists

The general consensus among those people who allegedly know reality, like philosophers and scientists, is that reality is just out of reach for normal people. Sellars' (1962) distinction between manifest and the scientific image captures this. Experientially stuck in the manifest image, we learned to believe that reality is captured by the scientific image, something populated by unimaginable entities like quarks but at least based on a solid mix of evidence and math, while we all know that the manifest image is a complete illusion.

Neuroscience has its way of explaining this situation. For example, Hoffman (2020) and Seth (2021) argue that all of our experiences are but a constrained hallucination. A kind of dreaming that is not completely arbitrary but mediated by sensory input and thus able to function like a user interface on a modern computer. Such a UI gives us visual representations of, for example, files that allow us to manipulate them by dragging and dropping them from one folder to another, without any need for an actual resemblance between the file on screen and the actual file in the computer as an electronically encoded sequence of ones and zeroes. Ones and zeroes that themselves are representing maybe a picture of a text in an old book again without any actual resemblance of that text but providing a functional connection that allows programs to display that page on the screen in a way that makes our eyes experience it as if it was in front of them. Nothing is what it seems, and yet it somehow works.

The hope though that Sellars' scientific image could rescue access to a real world is also in vain. As Cassirer (2010) showed already in 1929 in his analysis of the phenomenology of cognition, there is no hope to gain true reality via scientific analysis either, because every scientific insight is shaped by the conceptual formulation of the question. We have an endless regress of symbolic systems influencing what is capable of being described and captured by them, i.e. whatever our symbolic system we use to capture the scientific image will taint and colour that image. If we describe the world through the lens of nuclear physics, it will look different than when we describe it through the lens of chemistry or biology. All descriptions of the world are interpretations piled on top of interpretations – conceptual systems that can be exchanged with other humans and that become part of the great social process of the creation of what we usually call objective reality.

Science is just another part of that reality. A social team sport, thousands of brains engage in a process of running experiments and discussing their results and their interpretations in order to come up with mutually constrained, refined, checked and tested stories describing the collective controlled experiences, allowing us to predict the outcomes of their experiments. The scientific image emerging is not objective reality but an abstract construction coproduced by the community of scientists. Hallucinating together but using their collective processes to refine a system of ideas. That so-called objective reality is a social construct but not an arbitrary illusion. It has its advantages, it works for some things, and it allows us to create machines that allow us to fly over oceans and medicine to cure most illnesses and build tall buildings that allow us to live in the clouds. But none of these things can give us a sense of our reality that could completely liberate us from that uncanny feeling. The sense of something unresolved or unreachable. That there is always something that goes beyond what can be made sense of by symbolic systems.

The affective turn

The affective turn, as documented, for example, in Gregg and Seigworth (2010), happened in the 1990 when the linguistic turn fizzled out among analytic and continental philosophers alike. Theory discovered the body and the raw experience reevaluating and rediscovering thinkers who had prepared the ground. For example, Massumi (2002) reappraises the ideas about affect from Deleuze and Guattari; Eve Kosowski Sedgwick and Adam Frank's *Shame and Her Sisters* (1995), picking up on Silvan Tomkins' (2008) theories about affect as a basic operating system for humans. When it comes to talking about affect and affect theory, one has to acknowledge that there are at least four quite distinct ways of approaching a theory of affect. Roughly speaking, they are the Deleuzian approach rooted in Spinoza (e.g. Deleuze and Guattari, 2004, 2013; Massumi, 2002), which treats affect as a general intensity which could be seen as independent of an individual subject, even traversing different subjects and thus potentially connecting them on pre-verbal pre-individual level.

While the Deleuzian stance renders affect as sub-subjective and pre-phenomenological, Michel Henry followed a hyper-subjective line in *The Essence of Manifestation* (1987) and fleshed it out further in his Material Phenomenology (2008), writing of affect as raw experience, as the experience of experience itself and as auto-affective sense of being alive.

While seemingly diametrical opposed to each other, they both differ starkly from Tomkins' (2008) approach that focuses on the identification of a finite set of basic affects (like joy, anger, shame, etc.) that seem to be biological in nature and universally observable in all humans.

His approach inspired Eve Sedgwick (Sedgwick and Frank, 1995) and others to their work in the field of critical theory by providing an alternative model of motivation and mutual human influence to the classic Freudian drive theory.

Finally, there are neurophysiological models going back to Wilhelm Wundt (1897/1998) using affect as a model for a generic nervous excitation that precedes any interpretation by the brain and thus provides a model of generalized emotions/feelings before they are interpreted within feeling concepts, thus allowing for models that research how people learn conceptual systems of emotions and how to apply them to their experience (e.g. Barrett, 2018).

It might be the sensible approach to accept that all these different conceptualizations of affect are rooted in different ontological frameworks and thus completely incompatible, and one has to choose one and then work within that frame.

However, I like to follow a different angle, thinking of different ontological framings basically as just different stories of how to make sense of something that goes beyond all stories. Not because it comes from a different transcendent realm but because it is part of a different mode of experiencing the world. The recognition of affect within each of those frames is always that there is something that can't be captured by the story, and each story always will just grasp in a partial way. For me the affective turn works as a general critique of the hope that was inherent in the linguistic turn, i.e. that if only we find the right way to talk about the world, all philosophical problems could be retired as nothing but unclear thinking. Rather than looking for the right story – the right ontological frame – we may follow the logic of mutual inclusion (Massumi, 2025) rather than the exclusion, with each of these distinct ways of looking at affect seen as complementary perspectives on the underlying flow of intensities.

We can relate the different perspectives on affect to each other by starting from a Deleuzian/Spinozian general view of intensities that meet in the body and see how from Henry's perspective these intensities give rise to how this body experiences itself as being affected. Tomkins' ideas of affect as categories of innate responses come then into play when we look at the body from a third-person observer perspective (as it is favoured by scientific approaches but as it is also presenting itself to us when we try to relate to what is happening with other people).

Finally, a neurophysiological approach to affect can be taken when we look now with a definitely scientific third-person perspective (potentially using some heavy measurement machinery, to trace neural activation) at what is happening in the nervous system of people when they are confronted with affecting stimuli in experimental conditions.

These perspectives are wildly different and provide different findings, yet they are all rooted in the same material world. They should ultimately be compatible with each other, as long as we take into account that we need to perform the necessary transpositions of perspectives.

All approaches fit within a view of radical immanence. For Henry, that immanence is the immanence of the auto-affective flesh of the living body, while for Deleuze, it is not tied to any sense of subjectivity but about processes within the plane of immanence. Tomkins and the neuroscientists are also coming from an angle of immanence, even though they wouldn't call it like that, since they are committed to a materialist scientific worldview.

What unites all the different approaches to affect is an *immanent naturalistic view* rather than a transcendent view of the world. They are all compatible with a general process view of humans as becomings or dynamic systems – a general attitude towards affect that we can find already in Nietzsche's notion of the will to power.

Immanent spirituality?

One could see these developments as pointers towards an immanent spirituality. A spirituality that has nothing to do with a spirit world or religious ideas about a transcendent realm of the spirits, nor the one spirit that Hegel saw developing in the collective workings of human minds. Instead, spirit refers to a characteristic of material reality that goes beyond discreet facts and simple causal chains of physical forces. Something that emerges from complex interactions of forces and then becomes some kind of power in itself. Something that powers human characters, or other complex events like a rock concert, or a protest march, or a political rally, a seance, etc.

This kind of affect-driven spirit could be thought of as an emergent phenomenon, the most clear and ubiquitous example of what we have in ourselves and our fellow human beings. A spirit that doesn't come from above but from below as it emerges out of the material structures that form us.

This reflects Gendlin's idea that the unconscious is the body and that the body is a source of information and innovation (Gendlin, 2003). Our conscious mind, by which we actually mean the train of thought, is just a symbolic conceptual commentary on the world, but there is a more complex reality, which is what gives us feelings and especially the feeling of being connected with something bigger and mysterious that seems to transcend the confines of the material world and is at heart the experience of the continuous complex nature of the material world that doesn't fit within the narrow narrative of the material world we usually avail ourselves of.

Our narratives are powerful tools to deal with the world, but they are always just a commentary on the richness of the full experience. In Zen and Psychoanalysis, Erich Fromm (1960/2013) considers the example of a child rolling a ball on a surface. For the child, this is a unique, marvellous experience. The child can do the same thing over and over again and each time marvel at it fresh, because it is a unique real experience rather than an abstract description of a ball rolling across the surface. Language reduces the richness of the experience to simple repetition. At the same time, it gives us the ability to see a ball as an object, and in that sense, language is a powerful tool allowing us to create an objective world with all the possibilities that this opens up. However, we need to remember that it is not the real world. And that what gives that world and the things within it meaning is not the linguistic structure or semantic rules but the connection with the lived experience, i.e. *affect*.

What is it good for?

Eve Kosofsky Sedgwick and Adam Frank (1995) wrote about the joy of reading Silvan Tomkins. What made their discovery joyful is that Tomkins' model of affect provided a subtle alternative to two overused models of human motivation. The rather inflexible Freudian drive model and the rather abstract model of the "repressive hypothesis" behind a lot of Foucault-inspired theorizing.

Rather than drives which are defined by outcomes (to breathe, breed, eat, etc.), affects in Tomkins' systems are emotions that are flexible and can be tied to any object. They thus allow us to delve into idiosyncratic expressions of basic motivations which can be shaped and affected by personal history or/and social conditioning, therefore providing infinitely more flexible and nuanced tools to approach the unique motivational structures of individuals.

Tomkins writes:

> unlike the drives, affective amplification is indifferent to means-end difference. It is enjoyable to enjoy. It is exciting to be excited. It is terrorizing to be terrorized and angering to be angered. Affect is self-validating with or without any further referent. It is these specifications that make affect theory such a useful site for resistance to teleological presumptions of many sorts historically embedded in the disciplines of psychology
>
> (Sedgwick and Frank, 1995, p. 7)

The model of the repressive hypothesis, on the other hand, leads people down garden paths of generating critical insights which get stuck in diagnosing naturalistic or essentialist attitudes in cultural artefacts and judging them along a hegemonic versus subversive binary:

> The 'subversive vs. hegemonic' structure of inquiry requires wholesale reification of the status quo. One's relation to it becomes reactive, like that of a consumer, accepting or refusing this or that manifestation of it
>
> (Sedgwick and Frank, 1995, p. 25)

If we seem stuck in a relativistic battle of narratives where power is the only decisive factor, affect can add an emotional grounding. It becomes possible to ask whether a narrative works or not. Independently of its internal logic or the power structures it references. A story can feel true or not. It can shift an emotion or not. This can be eye-opening in therapy when a client proficient in spinning up endless new versions of what is going on for them can feel the shift in their felt sense when a story actually fits (cf., e.g. Gendlin, 2003, 1997).

Gendlin's effort (1997) is on the whole about the recognition that feelings and emotions are a touchstone that is indispensable to understanding meaning. While it is maybe not enough to fully overcome solipsism, it is nonetheless the sense of being that comes with a direct affective experience of the world that allows us to make peace with the assumption that there must be an outside world.

While Husserl's hope that a phenomenological analysis could lead us to a recognition of transcendental essences might have been in vain, phenomena do give us direct information about the world. This might not allow us to deduce the true essences, but direct experience gives us feedback about the world.

When an apple falls from a tree and hits you on the head or we stumble and fall to the ground, then this comes with a direct experience that shows that gravity is more than just a theory. There is something happening that has a predictable impact on us that we can feel. Our experience doesn't give a simple true picture of nature out there, but it gives us something that allows us to distinguish between stories that work and stories that don't work. And while that might not feel like a lot, it might be enough.

Stuck in pure experience

Which brings us back to the trouble with reality. There is no truth. No final ground of being which gives us a firm foundation to stand on. Everything is just experience. The idea that we could establish the truth by comparing the experience to the reality out there is an illusion, because our idea of what is out there is always just another experience.

William James sketched out that problem quite elegantly more than a 100 years ago:

> The central point of the pure-experience theory is that 'outer' and 'inner' are names for two groups into which we sort experiences according to the way in which they act upon their neighbors
>
> (James, 1912, p. 82)

There are no ideas nor facts in the world that are given to us independently.

> There is no thought-stuff different from thing-stuff (...) but the same identical piece of 'pure experience' (...) can stand alternately for a 'fact of consciousness' or for a physical reality
>
> (James, 1912, p. 81)

> Though one part of our experience may lean upon another part to make it what it is in any one of several aspects in which it may be considered, experience as a whole is self-containing and leans on nothing.
>
> (James, 1912, p. 113)

Whatever we experience, however we describe it, it is really always just another experience. What makes it at all possible to make sense of a situation is that we have different experiences that seem to correlate and connect. This is all that is necessary because we can use that to come up with ways to make sense of different experiences. A visual experience works together with a thought experience; to think, "this is a stone", works together with the experience of kicking it, with a sensation experience.

Connecting different experiences to create a complex image of how the world works is a complex process. Many of those combinations are also happening within the body before we are aware of it, what is called sensory integration. The McGurk effect (McGurk and MacDonald, 1976) shows how something as basic as the experience of sound and vision is already interpretations. People being played the audio for "pa" while seeing a film of someone mouthing "ka" actually experience hearing "ta". I.e. the acoustic event that they experience is not purely based on the sounds but is already the result of their brain mixing the acoustic and visual information and creating a reasonable interpretation for the divergent sensory signals.

There is arguably a constant struggle in our fields of experience where we try to find sensible interpretations for different experiences that either co-occur or follow each other in more or less predictable ways. Like the pain in the toe that may occur when we kick a stone. These are all different affects that bounce off each other and give rise to new affects within us, when, for example, a pleasant experience gives rise to joy or a confusing mismatch of experiences gives rise to irritation and anxiety. There is no way to test the truth of experiences, but there is a sense of truthfulness or realness and that comes with consistency.

Congruence

Congruence is a key concept of the person-centred approach and one of the most valuable aspects of the theoretic legacy of Carl Rogers. He used the term originally in *Client Centred-Therapy* (Rogers, 1951) in two key chapters: *The process of therapy* and *A theory of personality and behaviour*. The basic idea behind congruence was that the clients suffered when there was a mismatch between their experiences, specifically their self-concept and their direct experience of themselves. When concepts and experience align, it is called congruence, when there is a mismatch, it is incongruence. Most intriguingly, Rogers went on to use that simple idea of incongruence as defining aspect of what he considered mental health concerns. Only in the following years, he makes the connection that counsellors genuineness and authenticity are indeed a form of congruence, and thus the simplest way to describe the core of Rogers' model of therapy becomes: *healing incongruence with congruence.*

If we were to sum up ideas from James and Rogers, we could say that congruence between experiences is what is at the heart of the experience of reality. When our ideas, actions and sensations fit together, that feels real. When they don't, that feels unreal and leads to worry and anxiety. The question is not if affect is real, reality is actually an affect.

Experiential reassurance of reality

One way to find congruence is by experimenting. Interacting with an environment, observing and learning how various actions, sensations and other experiences fit together. In a way that is the core of the scientific method. Science can be seen as the most general way to find congruence in our experience of the world. Interacting with the world strengthens our sense of reality, because we get feedback and this way of being in the world is a constant way of reassuring us about the world and reaffirming our sense of reality. Even if we find out that we are wrong about something that can help our sense of reality. The resistance that the world puts up with the stories we weave about it is the clearest and best set of clues to create better stories.

The most fragile aspect of our experience of reality is ourselves. We might have a strong sense of existing but how convincing is it really? In order to get an experiential sense of whatever we are we need to meet with another like us that can mirror our experience and in that give us a sense of our own reality. This is where therapy comes into play.

Therapy

The self is not a thing that sits inside us and that we could get a sense of by simply feeling it out. The idea that the self is a narrative seems to offer something to hold on to. It makes sense as a way to capture the complexity of our swirling experiences, thoughts, feelings. It might make sense to think that looking back at the end of my life that a long intricate novel might be the best way to grasp who I was. But that is still very different from thinking I *am* a story. The story is at best the vessel that can hold a simplified version of me for future generations, but that story is not the me who is alive here and now. *Affect is what reminds us that no story can ever be enough.* The experience of living goes deep and exposes us to a continuous complexity that leaves any storied interpretation like a thin film on the surface of reality.

Arguably, philosophers of the self-as-story are not really trying to convince anybody that they really exist as a narrative. For them, thinking about oneself as a story is more like a tool. Something to aim for. This is the character I want to be in the story of my life. As such, it can become a tool to design an ethical life. That still leaves us with the challenge of taking hold of our lives and trying to turn ourselves into that person we want to be. A challenge which acknowledges that this is not something given (e.g. it doesn't come preinstalled with the body) but something that is constructed, maintained, refined, curated, while also being open to outside influences, i.e. manipulated, confused, distorted, twisted by expectations, demands, conditions of worth, indoctrination, education, mutilation, force and temptation.

It can be a tough challenge, and arguably every person needs to find some way to meet it. And people do try to make the best of it. When people come into therapy, they are driven by a desire to figure out what's going on, and because they are always already deep into that struggle, they don't need someone to take charge of their situation and tell them who they really are but someone who supports them in figuring that out for themselves (Bohart and Kallman, 1999).

An explanation often given for that desire of the client to figure their life out and make the best of it is the actualizing tendency (Rogers, 1959). What is usually missed in that explanation is that the actualizing tendency is a *tendency*, i.e. something we can observe as a rule of thumb but not a force that makes things happen or motivates people. Clients are motivated by strong affects – the direct experience of anxiety, depression, panic, misery that reflect their inner struggle for congruence. Incongruence may be described as perceiving a set of chaotic experiences that don't fit together and feel unacceptable, because of the lack of matching explanatory experience or narrative that makes sense of them.

We want to be congruent because it feels good. We hate being incongruent because it makes us miserable. The key point about congruence is that it is not a given state. There is no rule on how to be congruent; there is no right or wrong way to be congruent. If we consider the original picture of everybody just being faced with a field of experiences, the challenge is to bring it into some kind of working order, but that order is not given by our "authentic core self" as designated at the beginning of time. The only thing that makes it appear is the subjective experience of it all making sense for the person experiencing it. In this sense, one could ask how anybody could possibly be helpful with that entirely subjective task of herding experiences that are only happening for the person in question.

While it is true that only the person can find that congruence because only they are in touch with the full picture, only they can know whether something works or not, it would be wrong to think they are entirely alone in this because as much as our experiences are not fully private.

When a therapist talks to a person in a welcoming and non-judgemental way, they allow the person to open up and interact with them in a way that creates an affective connection.

Affects can help us to see how. Fear, joy, anger are experienced and expressed in universally recognizable ways by all human beings independent of cultural background (although those experiences can be overlaid and modified by specific cultural context). A Japanese samurai will react differently to devastating news than a Brazilian housewife, but a teenager in England can watch movies about samurai's and telenovelas and relate to both their reactions.

What is at play here is what Rogers described as "What is most personal is most general". (1961, p. 26): the surprising realization that feelings of shame, fear and anger which might feel most private, once allowed to show can be recognized quite generally among human beings. Fromm describes how this ability to connect with what is assumed to be quite a private core can lead to deep sense of connection:

> If I perceive in another person mainly the surface, I perceive mainly the differences, that which separates us. If I penetrate to the core, I perceive our identity, the fact of our brotherhood. This relatedness from center to center - instead of that from periphery to periphery - is 'central relatedness'.
>
> (Fromm, 1956, p. 56)

It also makes sense to acknowledge the Deleuzian type of affects here as general intensities that traverse individual human beings and can fill the space between them. This doesn't just become obvious in the behaviour of masses which seem strangely coordinated in big events like football games, rock concerts or political rallies, but also in the intimate space of the counselling room.

This explains how it becomes possible that such a strange thing as two humans sitting together and just talking can create the atmosphere that allows clients to make profound leaps and changes in their inner experience of wholeness and congruence, resulting in the kind of symptom changes that are still largely incomprehensible to the people who try to tie them to individual intervention in measurable experimental conditions.

Rogers never pretended to have an explanation how therapy actually works but he found a way to reliably create the conditions that enable and allow to happen what was needed for therapy to work:

> I find that when I am closest to my inner, intuitive self, when I am somehow in touch with the unknown in me, when perhaps I am in a slightly altered state of consciousness, then whatever I do seems to be full of healing. Then, simply my presence is releasing and helpful to the other. There is nothing I can do to force this experience, but when I can relax and be close to the transcendental core of me, then I may behave in strange and impulsive ways in the relationship, ways which I cannot justify rationally, which have nothing to do with my thought processes. But these strange behaviors turn out to be right, in some odd way: it seems that my inner spirit has reached out and touched the inner spirit of the other. Our relationship transcends itself and becomes a part of something larger. Profound growth and healing and energy are present.
>
> (Rogers, 1980, pp. 133–134)

What Rogers is describing makes perfect sense as a state of being with and resonating with the client and their experience. This in turn allows the clients to feel real and see themselves reflected in a way that allows them to get in touch with their own process. We know that this environment is healing and the idea that the special caring and welcoming environment allows the clients to experiment with their experience of themselves in interaction. An environment that allows them to get the kind of honest and open feedback that allows them in their struggle for congruence.

Is this struggle for congruence confined to the inner life of an individual or does it apply, as I think it does to groups, couples, families, teams at work, crowds and whole societies? Affect is our way of responding to and feeling the material environment in which all these entities exist.

The hermeneutic struggle

The fundamental problem of the human experience of reality is that it doesn't come as a neat story or theory of how everything really is. It is a jumble of many experiences, sensations, thoughts, emotions. There is no central authorial voice that knows it all, that can sum it all up for us. This is not a bug but a feature, as the techies say, because, as affect teaches us, any symbolic attempt to represent reality misses a lot of what really matters.

And yet we cannot escape the conceptual symbolic world of narratives, how we plug into the bigger world of culture and society. At the point when we become aware of that world, we are always already in a world of language and the world of concepts that we inherit from our parents and siblings and the whole language community into which we are born. Affect is a guide, a grounding, but also a challenge to making sense of the narratives we are surrounded by.

The resulting struggle, what we might call the hermeneutic struggle to make sense of the experiential world, highlights an aspect of mental health concerns that often gets forgotten in the contemporary culture that is fixated on diagnosing and treating what is conceived as chemical imbalances or maladaptive thought and behavioural patterns. What we bring to therapy, as alien as it might feel to us, is usually embedded and arising out of every day experience. Anxiety and depression and other uncomfortable and extreme affective states are symptoms that can guide us in what is a normal part of life, i.e. that struggle to find congruence in the experiential and narrative interpretations of the streams of affects traversing our awareness at any moment.

Therapy cannot do the struggle for us but it can support us. It is a challenge every person has to meet for themselves because they alone are in touch with the fullness of their experiential world. Only we are able to take on that struggle and find congruent ways of bringing the strands of their experiential world together. However, we don't have to meet that challenge alone. The presence of a therapist and their congruent reflections can help as an additional touchstone and can help to bring into awareness what could otherwise may be overlooked, missed, denied or ignored. The more congruent the therapist, the clearer the reflection. The more empathic, the richer the feedback. Acceptance and warmth help to feel us held and keep our nerve in the depth of the struggle.

The goal is not perfect harmony because the life process and with it the struggle never stops, not even for what Rogers (1980) called the fully functioning person. What we can hope for is to learn to love the struggle. At least in those moments when we can feel that we are riding the crest of the experiential streams of narratives and affects coming together in some sense of a congruent reality. Then it can actually be a joy to make that hermeneutic struggle work.

So this is what we can hope for, what therapy is about, to enable people to embrace their struggle, their personal search for congruence and make their peace with that being an ongoing process that only feels stressful or painful when it is interrupted or blocked but can be invigorating when allowed to flow freely. Because then we can at least come close to feeling fully real: fully in touch with a reality as something lived.

References

Barrett, L. F. (2018) *How Emotions are Made: The Secret Life of the Brain.* London: Pan Books (electronic edition).

Bohart, A. C. and Tallman, K. (1999) *How Clients Make Therapy Work - The Process of Active Self-Healing.* Washington, DC: American Psychological Association.

Cassirer, E. (2010) *Philosophie der symbolischen Forme* (3 Vol). Hamburg: Meiner.

Clarke, A. C. (1972) *Report on Planet Three.* London: Gollancz.

Deleuze, G. and Guattari, F. (2004) *Anti-Oedipus - Capitalism and Schizophrenia,* trans. R. Hurley, M. Seem, and H. R. Lane. London: Continuum.
Deleuze, G. and Guattari, F. (2013) *A Thousand Plateaus.* London: Bloomsbury Academic.
Fromm, E. (1956) *The Art of Loving.* New York: Open Road.
Fromm, E. (1960/2013) *Psychoanalysis and Zen Buddhism.* New York: Open Road.
Gendlin, E. T. (1962/1997) *Experiencing and the Creation of Meaning - A Philosophical and Psychological Approach to the Subjective.* Evanston, IL: Northwestern University Press.
Gendlin, E. T. (2003) *Focusing: How to Gain Direct Access to Your Body's Knowledge* (25th Anniversary Edition). London: Rider (Random House).
Gregg, M. and Seigworth (eds.) (2010) *The Affect Theory Reader.* Durham, NC: Duke University Press.
Henry, M. (2008) *Material Phenomenology,* trans. S. Davidson. New York: Fordham University Press.
Hoffman, D. D. (2020) *The Case against Reality: How Evolution Hid the Truth from Our Eyes.* London: Penguin.
James, W. (1912) *Essays in Radical Empiricism.* New York: Longmans, Green and Co.
Massumi, B. (2002) *Parables for the Virtual - Movement, Affect, Sensation.* Durham, NC: Duke University Press, Kindle Edition.
Massumi, B. (2025) *The personality of Power: A theory for Anti-Fascist Life.* Durham, NC: Duke University Press.
McGurk, H. and MacDonald, J. (1976) Hearing lips and seeing voices. *Nature,* 264(5588): 746–748.
Rogers, C. R. (1951). *Client-centered therapy; its current practice, implications, and theory.* Boston, MA: Houghton Mifflin.
Rogers, C. R. (1961) *On Becoming a Person.* London: Constable.
Rogers, C. R. (1980) *A Way of Being.* London: Constable. Kindle Edition.
Sedgwick, E. K. and Frank, A. (1995) Shame in the Cybernetic Fold: Reading Silvan Tomkins. In: *Shame and Its Sisters: A Silvan Tomkins Reader,* E. K. Sedgwick and A. Frank (eds.). 1–28. Durham, NC: Duke University Press.
Sellars, W. (1962) Philosophy and the Scientific Image of Man. In: *Frontiers of Science and Philosophy,* R. Colodny (ed.). 35–78. Pittsburgh, PA: University of Pittsburgh Press.
Seth, A. (2021) *Being You: A New Science of Consciousness.* London: Faber & Faber.
Tomkins, S. S. (2008) *Affect Imagery Consciousness: The Complete Edition.* New York: Springer. Kindle edition.
Wundt, W. (1897/1998) *Outlines of Psychology,* trans. C. H. Judd. Bristol: Thoemmes Press.

Chapter 16

Affect in person-centred and focusing-oriented psychotherapy

Yannis Rigas

Affective states

Affect is the bodily capacity to affect and be affected through encounters. It is a felt modulation of forces, pre-rational and pre-personal, preceding language, categories, emotions, or sequential meaning (Massumi, 2002, p28). Affective states carry a preconscious intensity where action is suspended (Massumi, 2002, p106), initiating a bodily logic beyond intention, a strange intelligence that experiences transitions, thresholds, and mutations. Something in affective states is encountered only in instants — a shock, disorientation, glitch — a crossing of thresholds that resists naming but can be felt as a change. A "space-out" exemplifies this: eyes fixed on an empty scene, meaning evades us, while speech and body coordination dissolve. There is an interval, a freeze, an interruption, another sense of space and a strange way of temporalization (Massumi, 2002).

It is as though an invisible current took hold — nothing specific, yet it moves us entirely. These states are not mediated through conscious thought but unfold as excessive and immediate flows. They are real but not actualized — not bound to perception or sensory-motor schemes. *Immediation* occurs when mediation collapses, creating direct affective connections. Deleuze explains that our perceptual system is bound to solids, not to flows or aerial intensities: "we are doomed to solid perceptions" (Deleuze, 1982–1983). Western thought and language tend to resist the liquid, the indeterminate. Affective states thus open a different temporality and logic. They are not empty or chaotic, but rich in indeterminate potential. They expose the world not as a fixed set of meanings, but as a field of forces, intensities, and thresholds where something begins to take shape. It is in this "before" that bodies wander in new capacities. To avoid any misunderstanding, affect does not signify any purity of being. It is just the other side of a coin of signification, meaning, personalization, and rational logic, which, however, includes them; it is constituted in a before, processes and conditions through which something is formed constitute the genesis of forms.

DOI: 10.4324/9781003669906-17

What is happening within?

In a space of passion a seer wanders in time

Unlike the example of space-out that was used above, affective states are everyday events, every time there is a steep diminution or increase of light or noise, of a synchronization with a differentiated rhythm and rate; but our body-mind have learned somehow to "smooth down" these frequent micro-shocks (Massumi, 2021). The philosophy of Baruch Spinoza is a central reference of how affects works: affective apprehension eventuates when two bodies feel a common way of "functioning", an "affective attunement" of a common flow (Stern, in Massumi, 2005, p172; p239). The affective synchronization between two bodies offers some knowledge of something that this world is enduring, because it is a constituent element of both bodies. This is a *collective* change of the body-forces which is a feeling of another degree of power or aliveness: a joyful felt vitality. The capacity to bear another degree of power in a joyful life marks an increase of power. It is an adding or opening in the force of existing, while the opposite, the sad passions of asynchronized bodies, withhold the powers of life, the power to feel-apprehend-act differently.

In a Spinozian line, Gilles Deleuze retells a theory of affect that we study here as a mean to understand affect. In this Deleuzian rehearsal, the bodily experienced apprehension of Spinozian *common notions* that traverse the bodies and the world are named *singularities*, and this differential dynamic of Spizozian motion-and-rest is expressed as *intensity*. Force comes always in multiplicities and any change in these multiplicities is felt as a passage of change, a bodily affectivity. Affective emission is what art does, it tries to wage compounds of forces exerted in every direction; in music, for example, it can be achieved through a differential between noise-silence-sound, of tonalities; in painting through a differential between degrees of light, of colours, or/and a liquidity of forms as in Francis Bacon's paintings (Evens, 2005; Deleuze, 2003). These sounds-noise-silences, on their own, make an autonomous body, atmosphere and space-time, which is itself auto-affected and uses its own references, thus it is an auto-referential process. In his cinema lectures, Deleuze speaks of affect in a very helpful way:

> Affect is this feeling inside… when the body grasps itself from within… it feels something in itself…I feel within me… the pleasure of feeling oneself…when I have an affect, I don't know what to do, and I don't know what to perceive. I no longer know… I find movements begun, but not executed, the indication of a more or less useful decision, but not that constraint which precludes choice.
>
> (Deleuze, 1982–83, Lect. 1)

According to Deleuze, in this gap of sensory-motor scheme, this feeling or grasping from within is *self-perception*: a body creates time for itself (Massumi, 2002, p36). This slipping into a time is a feeling of duration within a time that never stops; it is continuous and in a state of waving, a flux of time and "the force of time is what makes a power of life increase or diminish" (Deleuze, 1983–84, Lect. 5). This feeling of duration lasts only an instant, so short that it happens all the time but usually without bothering perception. To feel duration causes all kinds of pain:

> [...]physical pain, moral pain, agonies of all kinds, even metaphysical...all the actions that we have not even isolated and that attack us and that will penetrate you. You are going to be a thousand times defenceless, and that is going to create affects, all that, to create affects, and what will the affect consist of? A desperate "tendency" since at that point, movement, you have sacrificed your mobility on one of your facets. As concerns this facet, your motor skills, that is, the other facet, can only provide the support of a tendency... A motor tendency is what is painful. What hurts is a motor tendency on a sensory nerve.
>
> (Deleuze, 1982–83, Lect. 3)

Affective states allow the body to perceive other things it hasn't sensed before as well as perceiving them in a new way. What Deleuze calls *affects* and *percepts* is what defines power. Similarly, according to Rolnik (2023, pp14–15):

> Percept and affects... are real...they refer to that which is alive, within us and outside of us. They constitute an experience of appreciation for our surroundings that is more subtle, that functions as an extra-cognitive mode...I prefer to call it 'body-knowing'...In this plane, the world effectively lives in our body, generating (in our bodies) embryos of other worlds. ... to honour life in its germinating potency

What I find interesting in this account is that affect is more than a matrix of perception, rather it is like affect adds to perception, opens perception into "new ordering", perceives more of the world, something that "increases the power to exist" (Deleuze, 1983–84, Lect. 5).The possible pain of a threshold is probably modified into joy "that makes as lighter" as Deleuze states to his students in relation to Nietzsche (Deleuze, 1983–84, Lect. 5).

This new "minimally human" perception of something in a stream of life is "too beautiful, it's intolerable", it is remarkable, it marks our existence, since it grasps something that years and years couldn't; There is no object nor "I", only a seer that glimpses something unbelievable, it coincides with an object through deleting and reshaping (Deleuze, 1983–84, Lect. 9).

The body creates time for itself. The temporality changed because the line of the circle of time broke and an infinite set of straight lines traverses the body, it is inserted into a durational time. Since there is not a time-circle as a centre to revolve around, *time is out of joint* and the measure of time is no longer a spatial movement of points in time and a "before" that precedes an "after" that follows: now movement depends on one and the same time line (Deleuze, 1983–84, Lect. 12). Bodies encounter the severe and excessive direct time with no rational, subjective, historic centre, they apprehend without any mediation through configurations or reference. Enduring affective states initiates something like a becoming-seer in time – a *virtual observer* for Massumi (2002, p51), "a seer in the movement of the world" (Deleuze,1983–84, Lect. 9). A seer in time wanders in *pure memory* and not in fantasy, not dreams or recollections. Why? Because these are already configurations, they have objects and actors; recollections are images of memory, while fantasy and dreams are combinations of what a subjected body has already experienced in life.

Before we have a glimpse of the seer wandering in pure memory, we will say some things about the status of space in affect. Our common sensory-motor space is a lived and experienced space in coordinates; there is one and single extended spatiality; it has obstacles and goals, actions and reactions of its actors, "...where tensions tend to be resolved" (Deleuze, 1983–84, Lect. 18). The spatiality during affective states is a variety of paradoxical spaces like empty spaces or topological spaces, spaces that, for example, are not connected anymore; there are only perspectives that are incessantly overlapping. This is an alive perspectivism wandering in spaces of passion, without acting in them since "you belong simultaneously in two disparate and yet neighbouring sets" (Deleuze, 1983–84, Lect. 22; Massumi, 2002, p61). Into these passionate spaces, a perspectivist seer wanders through a region of the past among sheets of memory, all the past is spread into sheets that coexist: this is what we mentioned above as *pure memory*. The seer settles or strides from one sheet to another.

> [F]rom time to time [the seer] finds a passionate sought and settles on one… it becomes embodied or it is actualized into an image of psychological or personological recollection, then again scans the rest of the sheet
>
> (Deleuze, 1983–84, Lect. 22).

This durational time and this passionate space make up a *crystal of time* (Guattari in Deleuze, 1983–84, Lect. 14).

A seer in front of the whole past and future

Such a crystallisable milieu in which "we" do not act, in a non-chronological time of each past in sheets, assumes a circuit of exchange. There is a circuit of exchange, a refrain, between an actual element and a virtual (spectral)one. They are both real. However, the actual element is in a curious position, since it no longer extends into another actual element, because it is cut off from motor; this is why instead of an actor there is a perspectivist seer. A mutual element takes over when an actual element gets into a circuit with a virtual one, the *sign-particles*, which interchanges between actual and virtual (Deleuze, 1983–84, Lect. 18). This is indeed a strange story and logic of superposition!

This mutual sign-particle consists of *the present that passes which tends into future, and the past that is preserved in time itself*; time in this Bergsonian sense only preserves the past and is not an agent of destruction, the past is much wider than recollection (Deleuze, 1983–84, Lect. 20; 21). What a seer encounters in a crystal is the present that passes which tends towards the future *and* the past that is preserved. The seer plunges into the event, since there is not a succession of many events in time of duration: "you can treat as a single event a period of your life, your whole life, several lives together, or ultimately the entire universe" (Deleuze, 1983–84, Lect. 22).

Maybe now we can begin to understand why there is this apprehension of something that somebody could not capture through the years: an event expands in the present in all its pasts and its spectral futures: What happens after my death? Am I gonna love and be loved again? I fear loneliness: examples of an event that expands in one and only line of time: dying, loving, fearing, solitude, and so on. The seer is in front of a "retrojection" of the whole past and a "projection" of the whole present-future of this loving or dying in a continuum. It carries unbearable beauty and pain touching on a metaphysical and existential pain. We are "defenceless...a desperate tendency since in that point you have sacrificed your mobility on one of your facets" (Deleuze, 1983–84, Lect. 21).

Three presents of an event are spread in front of the seer: a present of the present, a present of the past, a present of the future (Deleuze, 1983–84, Lect. 21).

Neuronal power and sign-particles

Affective processes do not use signification, recollection-images, rational logic, subject positions, because these are machines of reproduction, configurations; they are already too formed. What emerges instead are quasi-signs or sign-particles operating in a "molecular complementarily", not representing but pointing, suggesting, inviting, and activating (Deleuze, 1986, Lect. 10; Lazzarato, 2014). Signs do not signify but function only within shifting chains, much like an invented language of children. Signs mark us across our whole sense. Their movement is non-discursive, guided by abstract machines that a body uses to navigate and assemble semiosis. It is not interpretation but scanning, sensing and emitting intensity. Affect is thus *pathic*. "Pathic" here does not stand only as passive but also correlates with *pathos* or passion, so close to *pathology*.

My hypothesis about these strange sign-particles we are dealing with here is that they are semi-signs/semi-particles of passion. These sign-particles implicate and emit an intensive quantity. The condition is felt as intense because it is like a changing wave of passion. It is a fluctuation of a singular passion, a multiplicity of powers that cannot be explicated through a muscular movement but stay within the nervous system as a neuronal flow of energy. These passion-waves remain within the nervous system, sensed as internal movement, an intensity, a charging of a body. Sign-particles are scanned differentiations of intensities in the energy that loads the body. They scan for passion or appetite of body-life in itself, and they mark peaks in the dynamics of passion in different layers of space in all pasts and present-futures. These passional markings are "multireferential and polysemic" as Lazzarato argues (2014, p111), since they are in a state of flux and thus meet other bodies.

In sharing affective states with another body, a body feels within itself this immediate fluctuation, simultaneously detecting something in a pathic mode of apprehension (Watson, 2009, p132). We are maybe approaching, somehow, the *auto-affection* or *self-perception* mentioned earlier. Sign-particles are marks of an intensive dynamic and at the same time mark the whole body and its whole history. One body resounds to another or two bodies are synchronized by a shared fluctuation of a singular passion. To put it in another terms, combining Spinoza and the language of medicine: at least two neuronal networks are loading the same ratio of motion and rest, of speed and slowness. This shared feeling makes them apprehend something both within them and in common, something that loads the world, an adequate Spinozian knowledge, a slight addition in perspective and in movement of their bodily mode of living. It is a kind of apprehension, an embodied or felt knowledge, a collective sense, a transversal knowledge across bodies.

Ethics

Affective states mark a crossing. A threshold in the multiplicity of powers is reached and necessarily fulfilled. This fulfilment occurs as the affect enters an assemblage, realized in the moment a body feels its own charge and transformation (Deleuze, 1973–74, Lect. 2). Assemblages define bodies not through categories but through what affects they can bear, sustain, or transform. Rather than a categorization, this is an ethics of immanence. The Spinozian question. *What can a body do?* – becomes a practical tool for *defining a body by its current capacities, not its abstract identity*. It's not a matter of whether a person or an animal is something, but how they arrange their relationships, how they enter into affective assemblages. The question shifts from what one is, to how one acts and transforms — from essence to process. This doesn't erase difference but affirms singularity: how a person configures their present in relation to a possible future through the past. For example, someone isn't simply a "patient" based on diagnosis, but someone who is actively configuring relations, even through struggle. Ethics here is *experimental*: a cartography of the present tending towards possible becomings. It's not moral judgement but a practical process — what Deleuze *would* call *a science of affects*. Assemblages are themselves composed of affects, signs, and assemblages; they function as modulations of intensity. They are real not because they represent something but because they produce consistency — material, affective, and relational. They reorganize flows of forces and sensitivity.

Relations between affect and the assemblages they enter into contain a *description* of things in terms of affects (Deleuze, 1973–74, Lect. 1). Assemblages are transformations of affect, they are signs in the circulation of affects, they affect us because they have been programmed by them (Deleuze, 1973–74, Lect. 3). Assemblages are arrangements of connections with materials and they organize and weight their consistency. We have characterized *affects* as (micro)shocks, because passages of a ratio can be very intensive, but for some bodies, an intensity that is, for example, very low, maybe deem catastrophic, that's why somebody needs to feel-apprehend what ratios of intensity are capable of carrying (Deleuze, 1977, Lect. 1;1973–74, Lect. 2).

Affect in psychotherapy?

At first glance, affective states seem very obscure in psychotherapy practice, since most psychotherapeutic schools hold a primary role for intersubjective speech and dialogue, actual relations, mutual recognition, rationality, chains of signification and meaning, clearing the obfuscating feelings into well-ordered emotion/s. The most common psychotherapies can be categorized as verbal therapy, and their main target is to bring unconscious thoughts, feelings, automatic behaviours, into a conscious recognition, a self-reflection and control (Bazzano, 2023, pp46–52; Friedman, 2007, p109). Affect seems to be most relatable in forms of psychotherapy that include art, such as art-therapy, drama-therapy, music therapy, and dance therapy. In this part, we will try to approximate and translate affective processes into two psychotherapy practices. In particular, we will bring as close as possible aspects of Focusing Oriented Therapy (F.O.T.) and Person-Centred therapy (P.C.T.).

On affect, P.C.T., and F.O.T.

Earlier we looked at how this pathic passion risks being engulfed within an intensive threshold of pathology and pain by assuming its own time as a whole existence to apprehend its sense in/with/as the world. Translated within the frame of Person-Centred Theory, it resembles Rogers's "organismic" "Actualizing Tendency" (Moreno-López, 2018, p96), the embodied drive that strives the best it can in every condition to persist and to realize its potential "away of being predictable and towards an unpredictable creativity" (Rogers, 1980, p44).

P.C.T. involves staying with the client's symbolization of (words, meanings, emotions, gestures, etc.), in order to affirm its current links or configurations of relations, to empty its exclusivist links (linear explanations, interpretations, etc.) once again so to create a new chance of symbolizing the same relations in a different manner, capturing something more from the world. At first glance, P.C.T. might seem inconsistent with the concept of affect regarding the value of emotion during therapy practice. However, as Massumi clearly explicates, emotion is one side of affect, and the side of the things actualized by affective intensifications always contain ways to return back to their unactualized excess or potential "laying the conditions for a reset and restart" (Massumi, 2021, pxvi). This staying-with-a-person's symbolization can be seen as capable of "exhausting its series of meanings and its external interactions" (Massumi, 2021, pXXIII).This practice of exhausting the most accessible formed side (symbolization, emotion) for a wider and oscillating "feeling" (to bring in the scene the theory and practice of F.O.T.) allows a person to encounter the more unformed side of an effect of a symbol; the side of sense which regards a panoramic whole of a situation, of a relation. An exhaustion of a current symbolization leads somebody to arrive at and confront the end of its formed series or line.

This return in an autonomous organismic felt apprehension or creation of sense within this life marks, in a sense, an inevitable return to the liberated and liberating tendency of the body. This back and forth between already constructed configurations and a vague sense of a whole of a body's life is what Gendlin *zooms in* through his focusing practice. This tension of back and forth between already formed meaning and a free-flow sense is what Deleuze in his own account on affect terms as "intensities". I argue here that this tension is recognized in both Rogers and Gendlin, because, as we will see later on, both have to deal practically with the psychological phenomenon of *the return* of the other's reference, what Rogers calls external locus of evaluation.

Narrative and description in affect

Narration and description are central in psychotherapy. They are the primary means through which someone expresses their inner world, organizes experience, establishes meaning, and begins to articulate what bothers them or what they long for. In this framework, a person narrates from a sensory-motor logic: cause-effect chains, temporal sequences, roles, actions — a "truthful narration" in Deleuze's terms, which assumes coherence, logic, and objectivity (Deleuze, 1983–84, Lect. 2–3; 9).

However, affect introduces a break in this regime. It doesn't follow the logic of actors and events arranged linearly. It disturbs the coordinates of perception and disrupts the truth-modelling narration. The body becomes a seer, caught in a flow, disoriented by intensities. Time becomes durational, space becomes topological — not extended but folded, paradoxical. In affective states, narration is not directed towards coherence or resolution. It becomes pure description — of events, intensities, transitions, and singularities. It is this rain. This touch. The familiar becomes uncanny, charged with sensitivity. This kind of description does not separate object from perception. It arises when the sensory-motor scheme collapses, when movement no longer links perception to action. It no longer serves a decision or goal. Instead, it becomes a passage, an entrance into something that is still forming – a passionate object, a sign-particle.

In sensory-motor scheme, objects are supposed to be outside of the perception we have of them (a classic take on phenomenology). We narrate external things and situations in a way that we decide in their instances what happens and what doesn't happen. We suppose a causal link that effects what happens (Massumi,2002, p28). This kind of narration of a subject claims to say the truth, it is a *truthful narration* (Deleuze, 1983–84, Lect. 2; 3). Truthful narration is connected with an *organic description* of things and situations though which we discern the real from the imaginary, and objects from their description of them; we install all objects on the same plane and we pass from one object to another (Deleuze, 1983–84, Lect. 9). In perception-action, we discern the subject that enunciates and the subject of the statements, while consciousness is the only admitted psychic reality (Deleuze, 1983–84, Lect. 2). In sum, truthful narration and its associated kind of description model the truth. But things in life sometimes, their truth, come to be in oscillation as if to say "I know all these, I have thought about them all, we have discussed them here, together, but there is something else there still bothering me…".

When perception collapses, the wandering seer feels things in another way. There is no noblest path to follow, nothing that wants to know. At every circuit, the narration and description do not claim to be truth, but a description takes the position of a passionate movement. In affective states, we are not in a position to desire, decide, or discern between real and imaginary, truth, or artificial. Time is without a central subject, and space is not organized according to obstacles or means. It is a state of undecidability of "alternatives between layers of past and inexplicable distinctions between points of present" (Deleuze, 1983–1984, Lect. 22, translation modified). Something passes, something is just *giving* and reveals "more and more profound aspects" of a passionate object in this incessant creating and erasure of the object in the circuit, it is a kind of entrance, and "there are good and bad entrances" (Deleuze, 1983–84, Lect. 9; 21).

Given that all the roles of the past have been played and failed, there is a chance to create a new reality, "a great exit into life" (Deleuze, 1983–84, Lect. 21). It is a *pure description*, a discovery of an entrance that becomes a face, a city, a landscape – something common becomes singular: It is *this* rain. *This* touch – an entrance is discovered in the preserved past (not in recollection) that permits a new beginning (Deleuze, 1983–84, Lect. 21). This is a vibrant feeling of a singular quality in a specific spectrum. This coexistence of distinct regions of virtual pasts are nor psychological neither empirical, we do not have to decide between them. There lays the child *and* the adult "in relation to the present that it was…It does not need to be actualized" since the "pure past will never be present and the pure future has never been present" (Deleuze, 1983–84, Lect. 14; 19). In this originary time, we do not know who is speaking or what it is saying. It is a time when "from the possible comes the impossible… as if the past is not necessarily true" (Deleuze, 1983–84, Lect. 3). This pure description, which coincides with a passion-object or sign-particles, allows a level of freedom from a model of truth: passion and virtue take hold over things.

Any description of this kind forms strange relationships, a kind of free indirect discourse where the elements experimentally try new relationships among them. A kind of paradoxical logic which links unlinked elements, spaces, situations and which is traversed by a new and unknown logic of its own (Deleuze, 1983–84, Lect. 10).

One form and methodology of such logic is what it is called *rhizomatic* connections: things are linked up in terms of micro elements by unique transformations, a threshold becomes a metamorphosis of something into something else which is quite dissimilar; however, these heterogeneous elements are somehow neighbours, in a relation through a distance (Rigas & Kolyri, 2024). A rhizomatic description forms a network of things, situations, processes that at first glance do not make any sense; they might seem delirious when expressed and might activate in the psychotherapist's mind the "red flag" of a pathological unfolding, an evidence of a medical pathology, or just a scene where the patient is extremely lost and confused. Still, with these kinds of description, someone is trying to apprehend something or has already apprehended something unique by using an unknown logic which nevertheless applies; a sense is implied somewhere below content and statements.

Listening and responsiveness in affect

How a psychotherapist listens becomes a central issue in both P.C.T. and F.O.T., not as technique, but as a condition. It's how the psychotherapist becomes a vessel for congruence or a felt shift. Listening with unconditional positive regard and empathic understanding allows the person in therapy to affirm themselves, without interference — not to be corrected or interpreted, but accompanied (Rogers, 1980; Gendlin, 1964; 1990). The response in these practices mirrors the listening: not evaluative, but gently reflective. A therapist may repeat a phrase, not any phrase, but one that resonates — that seems to open more than it says. This reflection is a question without an answer, an invitation to dwell inside something still forming. It introduces a pause, an interval where logic, judgement, even time is suspended. The moment is magnified. A phrase like "this anger" or "this smile" becomes not a report, but an event — a singularity.

These moments invite the body to apprehend something from within — not as "I feel angry", but as this something felt in the body. In F.O.T., questions like "Can you feel it somewhere?" offer a turn away from abstraction towards a direct bodily sense. This bypasses imagination, identity, and symbolization. Gendlin proposes the term "kination" — not image, but movement-sensation (2018, pp111–113). Such practices shift the mode of time and space. Ordinary metrics collapse, giving way to affective duration and topological intensities. The person is invited to accompany, not interpret. The therapist doesn't intervene but walks beside the affect. This is not about explanation or insight, but allowing something unformed to find its own rhythm, to speak its own logic.

In this sense, affective listening functions like a micro-break in the dominant logic of therapy — the one that seeks origins, causes, and outcomes. Instead, the body is asked to "stay with" the vibration of a singular sensation. This bypasses the linear, discursive logic of self-narration and invites the impersonal, the "it" that speaks beyond the "I". A shift from "me and my emotions" to "something is happening here". What emerges is resonance. A word or gesture may suddenly feel "exactly right", not because it explains, but because it matches the body's sense of itself. This is what Gendlin calls a felt shift — a bodily process resuming where it had been blocked. It's not a solution but a re-entry into the flow of life, a reconfiguration of the body's relation to its world. F.O.T., more than P.C.T., approaches affect directly through this bodily channel. While P.C.T. affirms the person, F.O.T. affirms the impersonal: the it, the process, and the unnamed. This doesn't negate subjectivity, it widens it. The body becomes a field of resonance, traversed by intensities that do not belong to "me", but move through and mark me nonetheless. To listen with the body, to the body is to hold open a space for affect to speak. It allows a mode of responsiveness that welcomes what is not yet known, a pedagogy of affect, rooted in patience, accompaniment, and trust in the body's strange intelligence.

Does focusing touch affect?

In the theory of focusing the main concepts of processes of "felt sense" and "felt shift" are presented in quite similar vein with the concept of Deleuze's affect: they are bodily capacities; they carry a different logic of sense or apprehension apart from rationality and consciousness; they are distinct from personal emotions; they are immediate; and curry something new. In what follows, we will further unfold and link some of these characteristics, while we will explore whether sense can be said of something that is pre- or extra-personal, extra-individual, extra-symbolical, or eventful.

In felt sense, like in affective states, this body-feeling is too rich for expressing it in terms of separate and clear-cut emotions. Usually, at the beginning, the focuser scans their body for vague or unclear feelings, not clearly delineated, not yet symbolized (or signifying). This is a step that allows the focuser to clear up the mental space so as to feel from inside. One could argue that this clearing up is rather a de-personalization, de-rationalization and de-synchronization of metric time. Why? Because this attention leaves all three behind, while a feeling does not have common categories of I/others, objects/subjects, etc.

So, a body is currently feeling something somewhere, yet unformed. A "second" move in a focusing session includes an invitation to abstractly feel *the whole of it* of a problem through the right distance from it. This feeling marks a tendency, a yearning towards something. The first two steps, as presented in the guide for focusing by Gendlin (2023), begin this felt exploration that include a pause of action, of logical interpretation, and a sidelining of known intersubjective emotions: focusers wander and scan their body for vibrations like a seismographer (similar to the wanderer seer in affect). They are invited to either stay with the occurring vibration-sensory by listing the problems they encounter and leave their sense to select the one which comes forward. If this felt-sense is too much, too intensive, one is asked to take a right distance from it: neither too close to cause emotions, such as a threat (for the ego configurations) nor too far to become indifferent.

In focussing's first steps, the processes of "distancing" and "surrendering" are crucial. The search for a right distance allows one to delink causes from effects and invites a person to accompany the present bodily felt effects. The usual search of causal logic leads to speculative, rational or emotional associations that hunt for the "whys" and the reactions to these causes, while a focus on felt effects delinks the cause-effect circle and transforms the "whys" into "how". As we analysed earlier, the question of "how" uses a description of things. It is a signal of practical ethology, which is operating in the present and calling for acceptance with an affirmative gesture. In this sense, ethics is the science of focusing on the how a-relationship-with-something is formed and what this relationship produces as its effects. It is a pausing moment, let's say, of weighting only the consequences of a relation in terms of how it is felt in the body. The body is not a subject that feels, i.e., pride or insult, but it expresses feelings by opening words into a panoramic apprehension of them. It is akin to the body reappropriating language for itself, liberated by linguistic social contracts and functions. Usually these feelings are expressed in terms of *qualities* (Gendlin, 2018, p207) – again we encounter this other use of "pure" description. Gendlin, in a similar way to how Deleuze theorizes affective states, thinks of quantitative qualities as "the best entry to focusing" (2018, p213).

This summoned distance, gap, or interval, creates the conditions for the focuser to wonder between the body-sense towards something that "speaks itself" a condition that might bypass, at least for a while any of the following:

a existing and dominant signification or symbolization;
b inter/personological and subjective narration;
c metric time and the extended spatialization.

If we interpret this in terms of affect, we could say that this is exactly what Deleuze means by *subtraction*, this emptying of distinctive configurations (action in space, I-other, subject-object, time of clocks, etc.)– a subtraction that allows signs to liberate their existing movements and get into a nomadic flow.

A feeling of a body scan is always about something that causes this vibration, this felt sense, and it happens in the alive present of the focuser. This is definitely in line with the centrality of Deleuzian-Spinozian value of *encountering*: the actual encountering is always causing the virtual processes (Deleuze, 2007), and this "meeting" with something or someone exceeds the categories that we recognize a given reality. The body is open and exposed to a reality that this time *is giving* more of its experienced knowledge of it (affect does not confer to phenomenological descriptions or mere empirical facts). The body has stopped reacting to a reality, it started co-figuring a new reality of relation(s). In these terms, it is the body that "speaks", not the person in their intersubjective environment; it is no longer "me" nor the "other" in the encounter, but the extra-/pre-, or sub-personal ways of relation (or encountering the unconscious) between two bodies and not between two persons (or subjects).

This way of relation is a charge common to both neural networks (I would rather say whole-body network), a shared aliveness, a felt coexistence, and a shared sense (apprehension) of the way they are relating or co-pulsating. If the bodies cannot pulse in a common choreography, in a common rhythm of relation, then this feeling of, perhaps, loneliness in life leaves its wastewaters behind, marking the body and causing a variety of bad effects (in Spinoza "sad passions" (Deleuze, 1996, p46), in Nietzsche "reactive forces" such as *ressentiment* and "bad conscience" (Deleuze, 2002), in Deleuze & Guattari's "territorialization" (2000), in Rogers' "incongruence" (2007), in Gendlin's "stopped process" (2018, pp14–17). Exporting a common sense that traverses all these different symptomatologies, "bad affects" have to do with something needed which is not allowed to realize their potential.

Having in mind the unrealized potential and its mark in the body, we continue with a third focusing step that has to do with a wandering in the body that accompanies a bodily shift, with all the other operations left behind – logical analysis, narration of contexts, etc. (Gendlin, 2023, p75). There, by grasping a "widened" sign (a symbol in Gendlin's terminology), the body feels more relieved/relaxed, as if diving into a stream or "a memory" that had remained forgotten (Gendlin, 2023, p75). It is a stopped process that the body sense finally allows itself to pay attention to a pathic attention that it is not a given anymore, but a giving of its existence to itself. A stopped process became a blocked compound and now it returns, or, maybe in Deleuze's terms, a sign that stayed coded and trapped in series in a cyclical time in the extended space, trapped in fixed meaning: a given. Now, this sign makes again synapses with a cloud of quasi-signs/particles, starting an exchange in a multiplicity, starting again not as a compact block, but restarting its process in a multiplicity with other processes (what Gendlin calls felt shift).

We have now reached the forth step, when the focuser approaches the feeling by a handling-word (Gendlin, 2023, p75), while sensing the tendency within its own assemblage. This move echoes the wanderer of passions that allows the body to feel this singular feeling approaching it through a logic of a spectral quantities: *it is bright, but not that dazzling; an opened yellow close to white, but not white.* There are two sides here, the sign and the bodily feeling in front of the wanderer, that start to resonate, till the cloud of signs resounds that of the particles: the two meet but they do not subsume each other. The focuser checks again and again their world with this particular feeling.

Even though this move brings back things in coordinates, this description is operating, according to mere affective qualities. Why qualities often express these body feelings? Well, it might not be words of qualities, but a logic of qualities, a logic which apprehends things as fields, in spectrums: the logic of solids is substituted by a logic of intensities, of aerials and their pressures, degrees of the same quality. This spectral "same thing" is exactly, in my understanding, what "singularity" means in Deleuze: it is the greenness of the colour green, the "smileness" of the smile, etc.

In focusing, the focuser stays, or endures, with this resonance of the double symbol/feeling that the body senses that it rightfully expresses exactly its condition; this double somehow resounds the Deleuzian affect in a circuit of exchanges of this mutual element of sign-particle, the spectrality of the actual sign with its virtual sides, the potentialization within a perspectivism. These are very nice words, but words sometimes curry us into their own magic world. What is at stake here is that something, a pathos, a blocked pathos maybe, resumes its *necessary* processes. This recharging offers a new, a different, a fresh sense and feeling, something that remind us of the

Spinozian intuition of a joyful passion which accompanies a joyful encounter and by the same time with a new "sense" or apprehension of being of/in/as the world. This is a shift of sense, a shift of how the body feels its life coextensively with the world, in "a now" that cannot be measured, not because it is too short, but because it never stops. Concurrently, this recharging of a resuming process follows a discharging of a blockage, that is the reason why Gendlin repeats that the best sign is a feeling of relief and a sense of "exactly right" (Gendlin, 2023, p76).

To sense and feel something new, to be able to resume a stopped process, to multiply the sense of a sign or symbol in a new assemblage, to re-vitalize and de-petrify a body, to learn and attune with the apprehension of the body in its life among other bodies, as in affect and focusing processes, gives something fresh from the world, an enriched world. It is not by chance that after these steps Gendlin puts a seemingly redundant fifth focusing move: to receive whatever accompanied this shift; configurations of ego and self-attack sometimes ring the door when returning to the logic of subjective knowledge and atomized life. The felt shift, like in Deleuze's theorization of affect, does not have to do centrally with solutions, these may be offered after all, but with this feeling of aliveness; that a problem is shifted to a better position or changed at least in a mode that might offer something more of the whole world.

The theory of affect returns to the body its capacity to apprehend life-processes in a similar way that F.O.T. creates these conditions for the body to express and feel its presence while currying all its experiential life that is flowing towards an enduring time. A micro shift of how we, as bodies or embodiments, live our life and by the same time a shift in our sense/itivity of our life or, in affect's terms, the way we are being affected and affecting while living.

Conclusion: a pedagogy of affect

"Affect concerns the revaluation of values… Given the transindividual nature of affect… Freedom is the transindividual autonomy of the affective process to generate surprises…Freedom pertains not to the individual, but to process" (Massumi, 2002, pxlvi).

It could be argued that a common aspect of P.C.T., F.O.T., and (Deleuzean-inspired) affect theory, each in their own terms, confer a process that auto-perceives and auto-affects itself through re-symbolization and re-signification (during process *and* as an outcome of them). This auto-attention has therapeutic consequences such as auto-realization or auto-valuation in P.C.T. (by recognizing exogenous valorization), reflowing of frozen processes and re-sensing the body in F.O.T. (by feeling the bodily shifts), and feeling the body from within in affect (by a pathic surrendering to bodily effects). All three processes are activated through encounters, by enduring them up to their felt effects on somebody, an attention that results in multiple shifts of valuation, feeling, and apprehension of something new. They imply that something of the world needs to be apprehended, sensed, and valued again: a transvaluation through a transindividuation, as Bazzano would have it (2019, 2025).

This kind of release or liberation of a body-mind from current constructions, invoked by all three theories and practices, has an effect on a creative being-a-person (in Rogers), a shifting person (in Gendlin) and a spectral becoming (in Deleuze). This pathic apprehension is a kind of knowledge through "existential transference" in Guattarian terms (Watson, 2009, p132). Some results of these three deliberating processes are at once capable of affecting the life-values of someone, of revitalizing their embodiment, of fostering creative action, of widening their perception, in sum, of activating modes of relating as whole entities.

If, as this paper extrapolates, affect can be brought close to the "actualizing tendency" in P.C.T. and "body felt sense and shift" in F.O.T., as well as their therapeutic conditions analysed earlier, then they already allow "multireferential and polysemic ... irrational elements" (Lazzarato, 2014, p111) and unknown feelings to unfold their own affective processes.

What I find most intriguing here is that P.C.T. and F.O.T. seem to offer conditions, or an environment, which might allow affect to be explored in a conscious way: a pedagogy and a therapy through affect or an ethics of affect. The proposal for "a conscious way" might be perceived from a rigid understanding of a Deleuzian perspective as inconsistent. In response to that, I conclude with a question: is there something more experimental and creative than a subject that practices ways of undoing its subjection?

Bibliography

Bazzano, M. 2019. *Nietzsche and Psychotherapy*. Abingdon, OX: Routledge.

Bazzano, M. 2023. *Subversion and Desire. Pathways to Transindividuation*. Abingdon, OX: Routledge.

Bazzano, M. 2025. On Transindividuation. Or: How can we overcome the enduring split between individuals and society? *European Journal of Psychotherapy & Counselling*, Vol 27, pp. 1–14. https://doi.org/10.1080/13642537.2024.2403433 [Accessed 23/02/2025].

Deleuze, G. 1973–1974. 'On Anti-Oedipus III', Lectures 01; 02; 03, University of Paris, Paris, 03 December 1973; 14 January 1974; 21 January 1974. Available at: https://deleuze.cla.purdue.edu/seminar/anti-oedipus-iii/ [Accessed 28/11/2024].

Deleuze, G. 1977. 'On A Thousand Plateaus II: Two Forms of Segmentarities', Lecture 01, University of Paris, Paris, 15 February, 1977. Available at: https://deleuze.cla.purdue.edu/seminar/a-thousand-plateaus-ii-two-forms-of-segmentarities/ [Accessed 28/11/2024].

Deleuze, G. 1982–1983. 'Seminar on Cinema: Classification of Signs and Time', Lectures:01; 02; 03, University of Paris, Paris, 02; 23; 30 November, 1982. Available at: https://deleuze.cla.purdue.edu/seminar/cinema-the-classification-of-signs-and-time/ [Accessed 28/11/2024].

Deleuze, G. 1983–1984. 'Cinema, Truth and Time: The Falsifier'. Lectures: 05; 07; 09; 10; 12; 13; 14; 15; 17; 18; 19; 20; 21; 22; University of Paris, Paris,13 December (1983), 10 January (1984), 24 January (1984), 31 January (1984), 28 February (1984), March 13 (1984) , 20 March (1984), 27 March (1984), 24 April (1984), 15 May (1984), May 22, (1984), May 29 (1984), 05 June (1984), 12 June (1984). Available at: https://deleuze.cla.purdue.edu/seminar/cinema-truth-and-time-the-falsifier/ [Accessed 28/11/2024].

Deleuze, G. 1986. 'Seminar on Foucault, 1985–1986', 'Part II: Power', Lecture 10, University of Paris, Paris, 14 January 1986. Available at: https://deleuze.cla.purdue.edu/seminar/foucault/ [Accessed 28/11/2024].

Deleuze, G. 1996. *Σπινόζα, Πρακτική Φιλοσοφία*. Athens: Νήσος.

Deleuze, G. 2002. *Nietzsche and Philosophy*. London; New York: Continuum.

Deleuze, G. 2003. *Francis Bacon: The logic of Sensation*. London; New York: Continuum.

Deleuze, G. 2007. *Dialogues II, Gilles Deleuze and Claire Parnet*. New York: Columbia University Press.

Deleuze, G. & Guattari, F. 1987. *A Thousand Plateaus. Capitalism and Schizophrenia*, Vol. 2, Minneapolis; London: University of Minnesota Press.

Deleuze, G. & Guattari, F. 2000. *Anti-Oedipus. Capitalism and Schizophrenia*, Vol. 1, Minneapolis: University of Minnesota Press.

Evens, A. 2005. *Sound Ideas. Music, Machines, and Experience*. Minneapolis; London: University of Minnesota Press.

Friedman, N. 2007. *Focusing-Oriented Therapy*. New York: iUniverse.

Gendlin, T. E. 1964. A theory of personality change. In P. Worchel & D. Byrne (Eds.), *Personality Change*. New York: John Wiley & Sons. Available at: Fromhttps://www.focusing.org/gendlin/docs/gol_2145.html. [Accessed 01/12/2024].

Gendlin, T. E. 1990. The small steps of the therapy process: How they come and how to help them come. In G. Lietaer, J. Rombauts & R. Van Balen (Eds.), *Client-Centered and Experiential Psychotherapy in the Nineties,* pp. 205–224. Leuven: Leuven University Press. From https://www.focusing.org/gendlin/docs/gol_2110.html [Accessed 01/12/2024].

Gendlin, T. E. 2018. *A Process Model*. Evanston, IL: Northwestern University Press.

Lazzarato, M. 2006. *"Semiotic Pluralism" and the New Government of Signs. Homage to Félix Guattari.* Available at: https://transversal.at/transversal/0107/lazzarato/en [Accessed 28/11/2024].

Lazzarato, M. 2014. *Signs and Machines. Capitalism and the Production of Subjectivity*. Los Angeles: semiotext(e).

Massumi, B. 2002. *Parables of the Virtual Movement*. Durham, NC; London: Duke University Press.

Massumi, B. 2015. *Ontopower. War, Powers, and the State of Perception*. Durham, NC; London: Duke University Press.

Massumi, B. 2021. *Parables of the Virtual Movement*. Durham, NC; London: Duke University Press.

Moreno-López, S. 2018. Actualizing tendency, organismic wisdom and understandingthe world. In M. Bazzano (Ed.), *Re-Visioning Person-Centred Therapy: Theory and Practice of a Radical Paradigm*. Abingdon, OX: Routledge, pp 93–109.

O'Sullivan, S. 2012. *On the Production of Subjectivity. Five Diagrams of the Finite-Infinite Relation*. London: Palgrave-Macmillan.

Rigas, I. & Kolyri, C. 2024. 'Ρίζωμα' (in Greek). In: Kesissoglou, Georgos & Maki, Kostoula(eds), ΑστερισμοίΕννοιών. Available at: https://conceptsarchive.substack.com/p/eee [Accessed 28/11/2024].

Rogers, C. 1980. *A Way of Being*. Boston: Houghton Mifflin Company.

Rogers, C. 2007. The necessary and sufficient conditions of therapeutic personality change. *Psychotherapy, Research, Practice, Training*, Vol. 44, No. 3, pp. 240–248.

Rolnik, S. 2023. *Spheres of Insurrection, Notes on Decolonizing the Unconscious*. Cambridge: Polity Press.

Watson, J. 2009. *Guattari's Diagrammatic Thought. Writing between Lacan and Deleuze*. London; New York: Continuum.

Chapter 17

On affect-based supervision

Manu Bazzano

The consolations of identity

To own one's sense of agency; to value one's own sense of belonging; to cherish subjective experience – these are important aspects linked to a basic notion of identity. One could ask, however, whether we have gone too far in prizing identity, to the point where it has morphed into subjectivism, the shielding of me and mine – my feelings, my emotions, my perception, my group and so forth – at the expense of shared values. If there is some truth in this, has therapy contributed to this situation? Initially, it helped us understand how crucial it is to own and express what is subjectively true. But the tide has turned, and we may have become incapable of seeing beyond our own backyard. Strands of humanistic psychology have historically been inclined to universalise subjective identity. But can subjective identity become a prison, particularly when it sings along to the blinkered tunes of nationalism? Or when it fails to be open to societal and political challenges?

Identity politics

In the public arena, this has resulted in the championing of identity politics at the expense of soulful solidarity. Writing about racial discrimination, the investigative journalist, Asad Haider (2018), defines identity politics as the neutralisation of movements against racial oppression, reflecting the replacement of socio-political movements with a docile multiculturalism. What once constituted a unitary front against the commodification and exploitation of human life in the name of profit for the few has now splintered into subgroups that cannot see past their particular experience. While it was once natural for a marginalised group to feel solidarity with another equally marginalised group, thus creating a united front of women, gays, blacks, trans, the poor and the disenfranchised, it is now customary to think and breathe within the confines of one's own group. To be a subject has come to mean to be subjugated to an existing order that defines my identity before I can begin to define myself. Identity is only partly what I choose. For the most part, it is assigned to and imposed on me by the 'Powers'.

DOI: 10.4324/9781003669906-18

Soul is a process

Anna, a transpersonal therapist, often mentions the word 'soul' when presenting her clinical work in supervision. One day, I asked her: 'What is soul?' 'Something you come into the world with. It is a divine spark that inhabits the body and travels on at the moment of death'. 'How does this idea help your work?' 'Intuition tells me whether a client lives according to her/his soul or whether this has been forgotten or neglected'. 'Is soul subject to change?' 'No. The body is, given that it is mechanical, perishable, and imperfect. But the soul is unchangeable'. I asked: 'Could the idea of something unchangeable be a consolation to a person struggling with our impermanent and unpredictable world? Is consolation enough? And: is this idea a belief?' 'Yes, it is a belief', she conceded, 'and as such, it is subject to change…' I believe this rather unusual conversation deepened our work, even though I do not share Anna's view of the soul. As I see it, notions of identity and/or an individual soul often end up being constrictive, while the notion of a collective soul is expansive. In one of Heraclitus' fragments, we read: 'It is impossible to discover the limits of the soul, or psyché, even if we travelled every road to do so – such is the depth of its meaning' (2018). For Heraclitus, soul cannot be individual; he questions the image of a separate entity. Instead, it encompasses the whole of nature and the world. This view found echoes in the 18th century, at the dawn of what was to become quantum physics. For the Jesuit priest, polymath and diplomat Boscovich, author of *Theory of Natural Philosophy* (2015), we must leave behind the idea of matter as indivisible, a symbol of which is the atom. This had consequences in philosophy. Nietzsche saw the idea of an indissoluble human soul as a remnant of this outmoded atomism. While honouring the ingenuity of the *soul hypothesis*, he went on to suggest new descriptions: the mortal soul and the soul as multiplicity of the subject; he speaks of soul as a social structure of the drives and emotions (Nietzsche, 1978). We may then consider soul on two interrelated levels. On an intrapsychic level, soul reflects the intrinsic multiplicity of what we call 'me'. This multiplicity is directly connected to the second aspect: the multiplicity of the world as a ground of natural forces. Both these aspects are characterised by what is essential to soul: its immediate link with transformation or metamorphosis (changing shape). *Psyché* (Greek for soul) means butterfly, a tangible symbol of transformation. A butterfly's life cycle is one of complete metamorphosis. In one of its three fundamental stages of growth (from caterpillar to chrysalis to butterfly), known as moulting, the caterpillar faces a tremendous challenge; it makes a new, larger skin and then sheds the old skin. From the point of view of the caterpillar, this process of transformation is disastrous. Its body is dissolving and a whole new being emerges after two weeks: the butterfly. This example is relevant to the human organism if one takes on board the fragility of growth and the tremendous amount of risk and adventure present within the process of actualisation. In this sense, soul is a process. This notion counters a view of identity/individual soul as static and separate.

Affect and vicarious trauma

At some point in his deeply humane and learned book, *When the Sun Bursts*, Christopher Bollas (2016) writes of a workshop he used to conduct in New York in the 1980s. I have adopted the exercise over the last few years in supervision group settings, with surprising results. In Bollas' workshop, therapists from various backgrounds meet in a group and discuss a clinical presentation, but the process is rather unconventional.

> The presenter was asked to eliminate all of his or her own comments and associations. No background information of any kind was to be provided; no history, no explanations of names mentioned, not even the patient's gender or age. All we would hear would be the stream of ideas, in the patient's words. Every few minutes I would stop the presenter and ask the group to associate. Interpretations were forbidden. Instead people were encouraged to offer associations from life, or feelings, or images, or to dwell on what might be evoked by individual words that struck them. We were not to ask the presenter questions of any kind, and when voicing our associations, we were to avoid looking at the presenter so that we would not be influenced by any facial expressions. While we were speaking, the presenter would take notes… Then we had the task of summing up what we thought we had thought… Then the presenter had half an hour to tell us about how what we had thought linked up to the case
>
> (Bollas, 2015, pp51–52)

The above example fosters a view of supervision that is not management, but open exploration. Bollas understands the above in terms of the unconscious; I understand it in terms of affect. Through being affected, therapist and supervisor can unfasten the artificial separateness of client-therapist-supervisor. That is when experience may be more genuinely accessed. This accessing of experience is soulful in the sense of allowing us to be affected within the shared domain of soul. For this to happen, we must reconsider the current professionalisation of supervision that has tended to present therapists' challenges as shortcomings. We must bracket our pathologising of suffering and reassess our need to protect ourselves. This is most evident when working with vicarious trauma. Zoë Krupka writes:

> The concept of vicarious trauma… cements the idea that some trauma… is surrogate or derivate experiencing and needs to be challenged through various means including compassion, reducing empathic connection and sometimes more physiologically distancing and buffering strategies… But why shouldn't we be traumatised by the brutalisation of others, either known or unknown to us? Why should our witness pain be pathologized in this way? Should we be protected from the impacts of forces that are much greater than the individual?
>
> (2018, p265)

Soul becomes more than a belief or an idea – it becomes tangible, provided we allow ourselves to be affected by our clients' suffering and our supervisees' own difficulties in dealing with that. What becomes clear, in the process of letting go of our parameters of isolation and exclusion, is that there exists a permeable, soulful area of experience.

References

Bollas, C. (2016). *When the Sun Bursts: The Enigma of Schizophrenia.* New Haven, CT: Yale University Press.

Boscovich, R.J. (2015). *Theory of Natural Philosophy.* London: Forgotten Books.

Haider, A. (2018). *Mistaken identity: Race and Class in the Age of Trump.* London & New York: Verso.

Heraclitus. (2018). *The Complete Fragments.* https://users..humboldt.edu/jwpowell/heraclitusTransBillHarris.pdf (accessed 12 November 2024)

Krupka, Z. (2018). Challenging Snoopervision: How can Person-centered Practitioners Offer New Alternatives to the Fracturing of the Person in the Supervisionelationship? In: Bazzano M., (ed). *Re-visioning Person-centred Therapy: Theory and Practice of a Radical Paradigm.* Abingdon, OX: Routledge, (pp 263–274).

Nietzsche, F. (1978). *Beyond Good and Evil.* London: Penguin.

Index

Note: Page numbers followed by "n" denote endnotes.